RECENT ADVANCES IN HEMATOLOGY RESEARCH

NEUTROPENIA

CAUSES, SIGNS, SYMPTOMS AND TREATMENT

RECENT ADVANCES IN HEMATOLOGY RESEARCH

Additional books in this series can be found on Nova's website under the Series tab.

Additional e-books in this series can be found on Nova's website under the e-book tab.

RECENT ADVANCES IN HEMATOLOGY RESEARCH

NEUTROPENIA

CAUSES, SIGNS, SYMPTOMS AND TREATMENT

MOJTABA AKHTARI
IHAB EL-HEMAIDI
AND
KAM NEWMAN
EDITORS

Nova Biomedical
New York

Library of Congress Cataloging-in-Publication Data

ISBN: 978-1-63482-105-6
Library of Congress Control Number: 2015931171

Published by Nova Science Publishers, Inc. † New York

Contents

Preface

Neutrophils are mature white blood cells which are the front line defence against infection, particularly bacterial and fungal infections. Neutropenia can be defined as abnormally decreased number of neutrophils in the peripheral blood. Clinicians started having better understanding about relationship between neutropenia and infection in mid-sixties and since then our knowledge has expanded considerably and a great deal of new insight and information have been obtained concerning different aspects of neutropenia including neutropenia in chemotherapy-treated patients. The authors have tried to offer an all-encompassing approach to the pathobiology and treatment of neutropenic disorders, and this book reviews current information concerning neutropenia. There have significant advances in medicine; however, bacterial infections continue to contribute significantly to morbidity and mortality in patients with neutropenia particularly cancer patients who develop chemotherapy-induced neutropenia. In this setting, it is important to understand pathophysiology of neutropenia and have a logical approach in diagnosis and treatment of neutropenia. Drug-induced neutropenia is another major clinical issue particularly in older patients which the authors have discussed it in this book. It is the authors hope that this book will help physicians, pharmacists, physician-assistants, nurse-practitioners and nurses to have good understanding of neutropenia and enable them to find strategies for identification of causes and optimal management of neutropenia in their patients. The authors have tried to provide an up-to-date synopsis of neutropenia in in the second decade of the second millennium.

Gathering all this information in one book will be of immense benefit for healthcare workers including physicians, pharmacists and nurses and this in turn will help them improve the care of their patients. It will also be of benefit for pharmacists are a source of clinical and pharmacological knowledge. For researchers undertaking research in the field of hemato-oncology or pharmacology this will be a useful starting point for reviewing the literature. Neutropenia is still being studied in patients in the clinic and laboratory models, and researchers are assessing neutropenia. The editors have tried to allow information in book chapters to show different aspects and various view points on related issues. The editors have tried to get all the permissions before publication, and great attention has been spent in the preparation of this book. Having said that, however, mistakes cannot always be avoided. The editors and the publisher cannot accept responsibility for any errors that inadvertently happened. The opinions and views expressed in this volume are those of the participating authors and do not reflect the views of the editors, the publisher, or the manufacturer pharmaceutical products named herein. We hope that our readers will find this book a useful and beneficial recourse in diagnosis and treatment of neutropenia.

Mojtaba Akhtari
Ihab ElHemaidi
Kam Newman

Contributors List

Mojtaba Akhtari Jane Anne Nohl Division of Hematology and Center for the Study of Blood Diseases, University of Southern California (USC)/Norris Cancer Center, USC University Hospital, Keck Medical Center of USC, 1441 Eastlake Avenue, Norris Topping Tower 3463, MC 9172, Los Angeles, CA 90033-9172, US

Kam Newman Rheumatology Program, National Institute of Arthritis, Musculoskeletal, and Skin disease (NIAMS)/NIH, Bethesda, MD, US

Ihab Elhemaidi Princess Noorah Oncology Center MBC-6447, King Abdulaziz Medical City-Western Region, National Guard Health Affairs, PO Box 9515, Jeddah 21423, Kingdom of Saudi Arabia

Wais Afzal Department of Internal Medicine, Jamaica Hospital Medical Center, 8900 Van Wyck Expressway, Jamaica, NY 11418, US

Mohammad Bagher Owlia Department of Internal Medicine, Shahid Sadoughi University of Medical Sciences, Yazd, Iran

Vijaya Raj Bhatt University of Nebraska Medical Center, 987680 Nebraska Medical Center, Omaha, NE, 68198-7680, US

Adrienne N. Nedved Department of Pharmacy, Mayo Hospital, Rochester, MN, US

Bryant England University of Nebraska Medical Center, 987680 Nebraska Medical Center, Omaha, NE, 68198-7680, US

Rajesh Shrestha Memorial Hospital of Rhode Island, Department of Internal Medicine, 111 Brewster St, Pawtucket, RI 02860, US

Srujitha Murukutla Staten Island University Hospital, Department of Internal Medicine, 475 Seaview Avenue, Staten Island, New York, 10305, US

Muniba Naqi Staten Island University Hospital, Department of Internal Medicine, 475 Seaview Avenue, Staten Island, New York, 10305, USA

Chien-Yuan Chen Department of Internal Medicine, National Taiwan University Hospital, Taipei, Taiwan, Division of Infectious Diseases, Department of Internal Medicine, National Taiwan University Hospital, 7 Chung-Shan South Road, Taipei 100, Taiwan

Ming-Shu Hsieh Department of Pathology, National Taiwan University Hospital, Taipei, Taiwan, Division of Infectious Diseases, Department of Internal Medicine, National Taiwan University Hospital, 7 Chung-Shan South Road, Taipei 100, Taiwan

Wang-Huei Sheng Department of Internal Medicine, National Taiwan University Hospital, Taipei, Taiwan, Division of Infectious Diseases, Department of Internal Medicine, National Taiwan University Hospital, 7 Chung-Shan South Road, Taipei 100, Taiwan

Samuel H. Poon 1Division of Rheumatology, Roger William Medical Center, and Providence Veterans Administration Medical Center, and Rhode Island Hospital and Warren Alpert School of Medicine at Brown University, Providence, RI 02905, US

Anthony M. Reginato Providence Veterans Administration Medical Center and Rhode Island Hospital and Warren Alpert School of Medicine at Brown University, Providence, RI 02905, US

Indryas Woldie Department of Oncology, Karmanos Cancer Center and Wayne State University School of Medicine, Wayne State University School of Medicine, 3990 John R- 3 Hudson, Detroit, MI 48201, US

Ayman O. Soubani Division of Pulmonary and Critical Care Service, Karmanos Cancer Center and Wayne State University School of Medicine, Wayne State University School of Medicine, 3990 John R- 3 Hudson, Detroit, MI 48201, US

In: Neutropenia
Editors: M. Akhtari et al.
ISBN: 978-1-63482-105-6

Chapter 1

A Practical Approach to Neutropenia

***Wais Afzal*[1], *Kam Newman*[2], *Ihab Elhemaidi*[3] and *Mojtaba Akhtari*[4]**

[1]Department of Internal Medicine,
Jamaica Hospital Medical Center, Jamaica, NY, US
[2]Rheumatology Program, National Institute of Arthritis,
Musculoskeletal, and Skin Disease (NIAMS)/NIH, Bethesda, MD, US
[3]Princess Noorah Oncology Center, King Abdulaziz Medical City-Western Region, National Guard Health Affairs,
Jeddah, Kingdom of Saudi Arabia
[4]Jane Anne Nohl Division of Hematology and Center for the Study of Blood Diseases, University of Southern California (USC)/
Norris Cancer Center, USC University Hospital,
Keck Medical Center of USC, Los Angeles, CA, US

Introduction

Generally, neutropenia is defined as neutrophils below1.5 x 10^9 cells/L. However neutrophil counts as low as 1.0 X 10^9 cells/L can be regarded as normal in individuals of African descent which indicates that ethnic origin of individuals could play a role in the normal neutrophil range [1]. Besides ethnicity, there are certain other factors such as age, sex, and smoking status which also influence neutrophil counts [2]. Thus, in any study of neutropenic patients, epidemiologic characteristics of the patients should be considered. Neutropenia is classified as mild (1.0 to 1.5 x 10^9 cells/L), moderate (0.5 to 1.0 x 10^9 cells/L) and severe ($\leq$ 0.5 x 10^9 cells/L). There is another term called agranulocytosis, which implies the reduced production of all granulocyte portion of bone marrow including neutrophils. In Agranulocytosis the neutrophil counts is lower than 100 cells/μL and is usually associated with dire consequences.

Obtaining a thorough medical history is the first step of approach to neutropenic patients which includes family history of similar condition, previous episodes of neutropenia or frequent infections, review of medications, and recent exposure to toxins and chemicals. Such a comprehensive history will provide the clinician with proper clue if one is presents On physical exam, neutropenic patients may present with fever, gingival, oral swelling and pain , perianal infections, skin abscesses, and at times severe infection e.g. a life threatening pneumonia or sepsis. If neutropenia is present as part of a broader clinical syndrome such as Felty's Syndrome then other features of such a condition may also accompany neutropenia. Neutropenia cause major issues as it can affect patient's lifestyle, as well as it being a huge burden on the economy considering the hospital stay, laboratory tests and other medical resources [3].

There are different classifications to describe the etiology of neutropenia. Neutropenia is classified into congenital and acquired variants. Acquired neutropenia is caused by immune neutropenia, drug-induced neutropenia and nonimmune chronic idiopathic neutropenia of adults [4]. Tables 1 and 2 present the most common causes of neutropenia along with their basic explanations. Each of the causes of neutropenia will be discussed in detail in the coming sections.

Table 1. Congenital neutropenic syndromes

Syndrome	Mode of Inheritance	Gene and Chromosomal Location	Clinical Features
Severe congenital neutropenia [4, 5, 6,]	Autosomal dominant	ELA2 (50%) (19q13.3)	Static neutropenia Possible progression to MDS and AML
	Autosomal dominant	GFI1 (rare) (1p22)	Static neutropenia Striking monocytosis Mild lymphopenia
	Autosomal dominant	G-CSFR (rare) (1p35.34.3)	G-CSF refractory neutropenia No documented progression to MDS or AML

Syndrome	Mode of Inheritance	Gene and Chromosomal Location	Clinical Features
	Autosomal recessive also known as Kostmann syndrome	HAX1 G6PC3 (0-30%) (1q21.3)	Static neutropenia No documented progression to MDS or AML Mostly in children of consanguineous parents
	X-linked	wASP (rare) (Xp11.22-Xp11.3)	Neutropenic variant of Wiskott-Aldrich syndrome
Hermansky Pudlak syndrome type 2 [7]	Autosomal recessive	AP3B1 (5q14.1)	Oculocutaneuous albinism Platelet dysfunction T-lymphocyte dysfuction Neutropenia
Chediak Higashi Syndrome [4,1]	Autosomal recessive	LYST (1q42.1-q42.2)	Neutropenia Oculocutanous albinism Giant lysosomes Platelet storage pool defect Lymphohistiocyte infiltration.
Barth Syndrome [4,1]	X-linked	TAZ (Xq28)	Neutropenia Dilated cardiomyopathy Methylgutaconic-aciduria
Cohen Syndrome [4]	Autosomal recessive	COH1 (8q22-q23)	Neutropenia Dysmophism Mental retardation
Cyclic Neutropenia [4, 8]	Autosomal dominant	ELA2 (19q13.3)	Alternate oscillation of neutrophils and monocytes with 21-day periodicity
Myelokathexis [1,9]	Autosomal dominant	Decreased bcl-x expression	Severe neutropenia Leukopenia
Glycogen storage disease type 1b [10. 11]	Autosomal recessive	G6PT(11q23)	Hypoglycemia Hyperlipidemia Hyperuricemia Growth retardation Colitis Neutropenia
Shwachman-Diamond syndrome [1,12]	Autosomal recessive	SBDS (7q11.22)	Intermittent neutropenia Exocrine pancreatic dificiency Growth failure Possible progression to MDS and AML

Table 2. Causes of acquired neutropenia

Autoimmune diseases- systemic lupus erythematosus (SLE), rheumatoid arthritis, Sjogren's syndrome etc.
Drugs- cytotoxic chemotherapy, chloramphenicol, penicillins etc.
Infections- HIV, hepatitis viruses, salmonella, rickettsia etc.
Sequestration-hypersplenism
Aplastic anemia

Table 2. (Continued)

Malignancies- leukemia, lymphoma, myelodesplasia, large granular lymphocyte leukemia, etc.
Nutritional deficiency- vitamin B12, folate, copper.
Irradiation
Granulomatous diseases- sarcoidosis

Epidemiology

Neutrophils are the most common type of leucocytes in peripheral blood. According to the definition of the National Cancer Institute the normal range starts at 1.5 x 10^9 cells/L which is thought to be the level required in order to protect against infections. Data collected between the 1999 to 2004 from National Health and Nutritional Examination (NHANES) clearly described the epidemiologic factors impact on the neutrophil counts [2,13].

Asymptomatic neutropenia has been documented in individuals of all ethnic background including Africans, Yemenite Jews, West Indian and certain Arabs but it seems to be more common in people from African descent [2, 13]. The NHANES study revealed that the black participants had lower neutrophil counts (0.83 x 10^9 cells/L; $P<0.001$) compared to their white counterparts, but similar lymphocyte counts. Whereas Mexican participants had slightly higher neutrophil counts (0.11 x 10^9 cells/L; $P= 0.026$) but higher lymphocyte counts [2]. The same study revealed that males are more likely to have neutropenia compared to their female counterparts within the same ethnic group. Considering the age, prevalence of neutropenia was highest in children younger than 5 years, lower during childhood and did reach the adult level by age 15 to 17 in females and by the age of 18 to 24 in males [2]. Finally, current smokers showed to have a higher neutrophil and leukocyte counts than those participants who never smoked [2].

In a case control study in the United Kingdom, the information and data retrieved from General Practice Research Database (GPRD) between1987 to 1999 revealed that women are more likely to get neutropenia, and that the incidence of neutropenia may increase among both men and women with age [14].

Table 3*. Mean Neutrophil Counts by Age, Sex, and Ethnicity

Sex and Age Group	Neutrophil Count x 10^9 cells/L		
	Blacks	Whites	Mexican Americans
Males < 18 y	2.9 (2.8- 3.0) P < 0.001	3.7 (3.5- 3.8)	3.9 (3.8- 3.9) P < 0.01 to <0.05
Males ≥ 18 y	3.5 (3.3- 3.6) P < 0.001	4.3 (4.3- 4.4)	4.3 (4.1- 4.4) P > 0.05
Females < 18 y	3.1 (3.0- 3.2) P < 0.001	4.0 (3.9- 4.1)	4.2 (4.1- 4.3) P < 0.001
Females ≥ 18 y	3.8 (3.7- 3.9) P < 0.001	4.5 (4.5- 4.6)	4.8 (4.7- 5.0) P ≤ 0.001 to < 0.01

* P values are compared with those of white participants.

Table 4. Comparative Mean of Neutrophil Counts in Smokers and Nonsmokers Age 20 years and Older

	Variable			
Neutrophil count, x 10^9 cells/L	Smokers	Nonsmokers	Mean difference between smokers and nonsmokers	P Value
Black	3.9 (3.8- 4.1)	3.4 (3.3- 3.5)	0.50 (0.3- 0.8)	<0.001
White	5.1 (4.9- 5.3)	4.2 (4.1- 4.3)	0.87 (0.7- 1.1)	<0.001
Mexican American	4.8 (4.5- 5.0)	4.4 (4.3- 4.5)	0.41 (0.2- 0.7)	0.002

Clinical Presentation

Neutropenic patients usually fall victims to microorganisms which are mostly components of the normal endogenous flora of body parts like mouth, oropharynx, gastrointestinal tract and skin. The severity of the patient's condition depends on the degree, onset, and duration of the neutropenia; severe and acute neutropenia most likely has a grave prognosis. A comprehensive medical history which includes patient's medication exposure, family history of similar condition, and personal history of recurrent fever and infections are fundamental to approach a correct diagnosis. Patients on chemotherapy regimen for malignancies or immunosuppressive treatment due to autoimmune disorders as well as patients with certain congenital neutrophil disorders are more prone to manifest neutropenic episodes. Medications such as thyroid antagonists, antibiotics or analgesics might be contributing factors to the in neutropenia and should be ruled out.

Patients with chronic and life-long neutropenia usually have less severe infection compared to the patients who are being treated with immunosuppressive or chemotherapy medications, [1]. The main reason for this is thought to be due to the effect of chemoptherapy on the host defensive frontier lines such as the mucosal barriers which covers inner portion of the body. For obvious reasons, the risk of bacterial and fungal infections is much higher if the etiology of neutropenia is bone marrow involvement rather than peripheral destruction of granulocytes [15].

Malaise, fever, mouth ulcerations and infection of the oropharynx, paranasal sinuses, middle ear, airways and lungs, bowel, perirectal area and skin are the universal presentation of neutropenic patients. On physical exam, signs of infection depend on the involved organ. Clinicians should look for inflammation and ulceration of the oral cavity, paranasal sinuses discharge and/or tenderness, added respiratory sounds, hepatosplenomegaly, lymphadenopathy or skin abscesses. The perianal region is a common place for abscess and should carefully be examined. Peripheral and central catheters are other common sites of infection in the inpatient setting and should not be missed. Hypotension and cardiopulmonary compromise are signs of septicemia suggestive of severe disease and are often associated with poor prognosis. The clinician should be aware that some other symptoms and signs can accompany neutropenia but are part of the underlying disorder. In Felty syndrome concomitant rheumatologic manifestation along with splenomegaly may also be present with neutropenia [16]. In cyclic neutropenia the clinical signs and symptoms are part of indolent course of the disorder [8].

Staphylococcus aureus, staphylococcus epidermidis, streptococci, enterococci, pseudomonas aeruginosa, Escherichia coli and other gram negative and gram positive bacteria are among the most common bacterial infections [15, 17]. Bacterial infection predominantly occurs in neutropenic patients during the early phase of neutropenic episode while in patients with severe and prolonged neutropenia or in those receiving multiple courses of broad-spectrum antibiotics fungal infections are generally more common. Among fungal infections Candida, Aspergillus, Zygomyces and Fusarium are the common causes of fungal infections in neutropenic patients [18]. Although viral infections are uncommon, herpes viruses (HSV, VZV, CMV, HHV type 6) and community acquired viruses (RSV, influenza virus, parainluenza virus, adenovirus) are the most common causes [18]. Overall, compared to non-neutropenic patients, symptoms of infections may be more atypical in neutropenic patients as neutropenic patients produce less inflammatory response to infections. Thus, pus and fluctuating abscesses may be less frequently encountered or absent [15]. Neutrophils have the diverse anti-infective properties of producing cytokine release, chemotaxis, phagocytosis, NAPDH oxidase and many other complex defensive properties and it is not surprising that neutropenia causes a profound state of immunodeficiency.

Workup

Starting with a thorough history taking and performing physical exam and basic laboratory examinations such as complete blood count (CBC) is the best initial approach. Before commencing a comprehensive expensive workup which could be costly for patients, healthcare institutions and insurance companies, some causes of neutropenia like medications and infections should be ruled out by meticulous history taking. If CBC indicates lower neutrophil count, it is advisable to repeat the test. As the name implies in cyclic neutropenia, serial blood counts are necessary to diagnose this disorder. In a case report, collecting blood in EDTA-contained tubes for laboratory assessment has falsely indicated neutropenia. Subsequent follow up with multiple investigational studies showed that ETDA present in the collecting tube caused leukoagglutination and pseudoneutropenia [19]. After documented neutropenia in at least two CBC reports, further investigation with differential count and peripheral smear for better assessment of neutropenia must be performed. Blood smear are one the most important labrotary tests which should not be underestimated as it will not only show a better picture of neutrophils but could lead the clinician to another contributing pathology like hematologic malignancy. It is also helpful to check vitamin B_{12} and folate levels at this stage of investigation. If fever and symptoms and signs of sepsis are present, appropriate cultures and infectious disease work up should be performed. Appropriate lifesaving antibiotic therapy must immediately initiated and treating physicians should not wait for the result of culture and sensitivity testing. Imaging studies like chest X-rays may reveal pulmonary infection secondary to compromised immune system of neutropenic patients. Certain viral studies like hepatitis B surface antigen (HBsAg), HCV antibody, HIV antibody and viral loads may also be helpful. In neutropenia secondary to hematologic malignancies or neutropenia due to hypersplenism and subsequent sequestration, abdominal ultrasound is an inexpensive tool which could be used to investigate whether splenomegaly is present or not. In very special cases, more sophisticated studies like abdominal CT scans may reveal some gastrointestinal complications of neutropenia.

Bone marrow aspiration and examination is often necessary to exclude malignant pathologies, elucidate cellularity and to asses myeloid maturation. Bone marrow examination may reveal certain neutrophilic syndromes such as maturation arrest in severe congenital neutropenia and large cytoplasmic granules in Chediak-Higashi syndrome [15]. Flow cytometry, immune-phenotyping, and cytogenetic analysis are some of the other investigations that can be performed on peripheral blood or marrow samples to establish the etiology of neutropenia. Cytogenetic analysis is the mainstay of the investigation and is of paramount significance in detecting congenital neutron-penic syndromes and malignancies.

Anti-neutrophil antibodies (ANA), antibodies against specific glycol-proteins of neutrophils, are very effective in diagnosing immune neutropenia. These antibodies are detected by several methods namely the granulocyte immunofluorescence test (GIFT), granulocyte indirect immunofluorescence test (GIIFT), granulocyte agglutination test (GAT), enzyme linked immune-assays (ELISA) and monoclonal antibody-specific immobilization of gran-ulocyte antigens (MAIGA). Among all of these different methods, GAT and GIFT are the most used [4, 20]. Neutrophil antibody testing has fallen out of favour oowing to the difficulty in its interpretation, and the presence of neutrophil receptors which could cause false negative results and finally fragility of neutrophils. All are factors which could make an unreliable test to utilize [4]. ANA antibodies are mainly IgG antibodies directed against certain neutrophil glycoprotein antigens like CD16 (FcϒRIIIb) and CD177, generally known as human neutrophil alloantigens (HNA) [4, 15, 20].

I. Congenial Neutropenic Syndromes

1. Severe Congenital Neutropenia

Severe congenital neutropenia (SCN) represents a heterogeneous group of genetic disorders characterized by absolute neutrophil counts below $0.5x10^9/L$ in peripheral blood on 3 separate occasions during the course of a 6 months clinical observations, early onset severe bacterial infection, and arrest of granulocytes at the promeylocyte/myeolocyte stage [5, 6]. It was first described as an autosomal recessive disorder by a Swedish researcher, *Rolf Kostmann* in 1956 [5]. Later, the ELA2 and X-linked wASP mutations were discovered one after the other. The most commonly involved genes in SCN are ELA2 (40-50% of cases), and HAX1 (0-30% of causes), while mutations in GFI1, wASP, G6PC3 and G-CSFR have been documented in smaller number of patients. Recently, simultaneous mutations of the above genes have also been described [5]. In spite of extensive investigations, the molecular basis of nearly 40% of SCN remains unanswered.

ELA2, also known as elastase neutrophil expressed (ELANE) mutation, induces ELANE-related neutropenia. It is has been recognized that the alteration in the gene encoding neutrophil elastase is inherited in an autosomal dominant fashion and is the gene responsible for SCN [21]. Neutrophil elastase is a myeloid cell-specific serine protease exhibiting pleiotropic functions by cleaving a wide range of bacterial and host proteins, explaining how patients with ELA2 mutations show decreased transcription and translation of neutrophil elastase and subsequent predisposition to developing infective syndromes. Besides infectious complications, patients with ELA2 mutations have higher rate of progression to MDS and AML.

Growth factor independence-1 (GFI1) is a zinc finger transcriptional repressor oncoprotein controlling hematopoietic stem cell differentiation by governing multiple target genes and regulatory microRNAs [21]. GFI1 mutation constitutes an extremely rare subtype of SCN and so far described only in small number of patients [26]. Caused by autosomal dominant mutation, GFI1 related SCN patients develop a triad of neutropenia, mild lymphopenia and a prominent monocytosis. [5]. Affected patients show myeloid maturation arrest, a paucity of mature neutrophils which make patients more prone to recurrent infections.

Extracellular G-CSF receptor defects, of which only 5 cases have been reported is clinically very similar to SCN due to ELA2 mutation and it is also inhereted in an autosomal dominant fashion. One of the characteristics of this disorder is its unresponsiveness to even high doses of G-CSF. A possible link between colony stimulating factor receptor (CSFR) mutation and mononsomy 7(q) has also been proposed [5].

Kostmann syndrome is a rare autosomal recessive form of SCN which is associated with HCLS-associated protein X-1 (HAX1) mutation. The antiapototic protein, HAX 1 is primarily located in mitochondria and maintains the inner mitochondrial membrane potential and thus protects myeloid cells from apoptosis [21]. Both hematopoietic and non-hematopoietic cells in HAX1 deficient patients are prone to induced dissipation on the inner mitochondrial membrane potential, leading to accelerated cell apoptosis and symptomatic neutropenia [15].

X-linked variant of congenital neutropenia is a rare type of SCN caused by gain-of-function mutations in Wiskott-Aldrich syndrome gene known as wASP [5, 21]. In primary immunodeficiency of Wiskott-Aldrich syndrome the same gene would lose function. wASP protein is associated with intracytoplasmic polymerization of actin, and mutation in this gene leads to increased actin polymerization and subsequent cell apoptosis [22]. Besides neutropenia, variable degrees of lymphopenia, monocytopenia, very low natural killer (NK) cell abrogated phagocyte activity and some risk of myelodysplasia are distinguishing features of this disease [5, 21].

SCN generally manifests as severe recurrent bouts of infections in the first months of life. Unless managed appropriately, patients suffering from SCN will develop chronic gingivitis, oral ulcers, skin abscesses, recurrent pneumonias and life-threatening septicemias [5]. The mainstay of therapy for SCN is reconstitution of sufficient level of host defense by means of increasing neutrophil counts with G-CSF in order to thwart any possible bacterial invasion. Appropriate antibiotic therapy will also be necessary in acute settings.

2. Hermansky Pudlak Syndrome Type 2

Hermansky Pudlak syndrome type 2 (HPS2) is an autosomal recessive disorder that arises from mutation in AP3B1 gene, which encodes the β3A subunit of the Adaptor Protein 3 (AP-3) complex [23]. AP3 is a cargo protein, responsible for packaging of intracellular vesicles (presumably lysosomes, melanosomes, and dense bodies) from the trans-Golgi network and endosomes in a clathrin-mediated fashion [7, 22]. HPS2 is clinically characterized by oculo-cutaneous albinism, platelet dysfunction and immunodeficiency arising from neutropenia and T-lymphocyte dysfunction [23]. G-CSF may raise neutrophil counts and and antibiotics will treat bacterial infections; however, other complications such as pulmonary fibrosis are typically symptomatic in the early thirties and can progress to death within a decade [7].

3. Chediak-Highashi Syndrome

Chediak-Highashi Syndrome (CHS) is a rare autosomal recessive disorder characterized by partial-oculocutaneous albinism, abnormal melanosome hair repartition, giant granules in neutrophils and other granule containing cells, bright red inclusions in some lymphocytes and NK cell dysfunction [22, 24]. The primary defect in CHS is attributed to vesicular trafficking defect secondary to enlarged granules in the lysosomes and melanosomes and platelet dense granules [25]. CHS patients suffer from nystagmus, photophobia, decreased visual acuity, recurrent skin and airway infections, immune defect due to impaired T-lymphocyte and NK cells cytolytic function, bleeding and neurologic manifestations. Finding of giant peroxidase in leukocytes, platelets, melanocytes, hepatocytes, renal tubular cells, and neural and thyroid tissue is suggestive of CHS, and finding the mutation in lysosomal trafficking regulator (LYST) gene on chromosome 1 confirms the diagnosis [25]. It has been shown that ascorbic acid (20mg/kg/dose) may correct CHS microtubular defects [24] whereas hematopoietic stem cell transplant (HSCT) is considered the treatment of choice to correct hematological and immunological complications. However, HSCT will not prevent the progressive neuropathy associated with this disease [26].

4. Barth Syndrome

Barth Syndrome is an X-linked disorder characterized by dilated cardiomyopathy, skeletal myopathy, growth retardation, 3-methylgutaconic aciduria and moderate to severe neutropenia. The primary gene defect in Barth syndrome is a mutation in tafazzin (TAZ) gene comprising 11 exons, which is located on Xq28 [27, 28]. TAZ encodes acyltransferase that catalyses the remodeling in mitochonderial membranes. A malfunctioning TAZ gene will lead to disrupted mitochondrial integrity and increased speed of cellular apoptosis. The management of symptomatic patient include increasing neutrophil count with G-CSF, proper prophylactic antibiotic therapy to tackle infections and appropriate cardiovascular care.

5. Cohen Syndrome

Cohen syndrome is an autosomal recessive disorder characterized by failure to thrive, mental retardation, microcephaly, facial abnormalities, myopia, pigmentary retinitis, truncal obesity, ligament laxity and neutropenia (90%) [29]. Cohen syndrome is caused by mutation of COH1 also known as VPS13B gene which is located on chromosome 8 and encodes for an endoplasmic reticulum protein [22]. From a hematologic standpoint, these patients are neutropenic, and prone to develop chronic infection. Administration of prophylactic G-CSF therapy is required to prevent the later complication [29] and antibiotics are only reserved for individuals with infections.

6. Cyclic Neutropenia

An autosomal dominant disorder, cyclic neutropenia is due to a mutation in the neutrophil elastase gene (ELA2 also known as ELANE) located on

19q13.3 and thus sharing a common genetic pattern with the autosomal variant of SCN. Although autosomal dominant variant of SCN also has the same ELA2 mutation as cyclic neutropenia, cyclic neutropenia does not increase the risk of leukemia or myelodysplasia in its victims [5]. What make this disease unique is that affected patients commonly have regular oscillations of peripheral blood neutrophil counts occurring at a frequency of every 21 days that lasts for 4-6 days. Because blood monocytes, reticulocytes, platelets, and lymphocytes oscillate with the same periodicity as blood neutrophils, the disease is also sometimes called periodic or cyclic hematopoiesis. Neutrophilic periods of cyclic neutropenia are accompanied by malaise, anorexia, fever, painful cervical lymphadenopathy (rather than generalized lymphadenopathy), and ulceration of the mucous membranes, both in the mouth and along the gastrointestinal tract [1,]. Affected pediatric patients are at particular risk for developing gangrene, bacteremia and septic shock. A diagnosis of cyclic neutropenia is established by obtaining serial differential leukocyte count at least 2-3 times per week for 6 weeks to observe at least 2 neutrophil nadirs [1, 5]. The regularly recurring neutropenic episodes and their accompanying infectious complications can have a lifelong impact on the patient's work, and social and psychological status. The availability of G-CSF has greatly altered the management of cyclic neutropenia, and has improved neutrophil oscillations, shortened the duration of neutropenia and decreased the frequency of neutropenic episodes.

7. Myelokathexis

Myelokathexis is a rare autosomal dominant congenital disorder that causes severe chronic leukopenia and neutropenia. In a case series of four patients the authors concluded that decreased expression of anti-apoptotic gene bcl-x may result in the accelerated apoptosis of bone marrow myeloid progenitor cells and participate in the peripheral neutropenia [1, 9]. Granulocyte hyperplasia in bone marrow and pycnotic nuclei of marrow and peripheral neutrophils are characteristic of this disease [1]. Similar to other congenital neutropenic syndromes, victims of myelokathexis are prone to develop recurrent infections. Infection with organisms of oropharynx, skin, and gastrointestinal tract are particularly more common and is often associated with substantial morbidity. G-CSF is used to improve neutrophil counts and decreased risk of infection.

8. Glycogen Storage Disease Type 1b

Glycogen storage disease type 1b is an autosomal recessive genetic disorder caused by mutation in glucose-6-phosphate transporter (G6PT) gene and results in glucose-6-phosphatase deficiency [30]. Located in the inner membrane of endoplasmic reticulum, this enzyme is responsible for transportation of glucose-6-phosphate from cytoplasm to the lumen of endoplasmic reticulum [11]. Loss of G6PT activity leads to enhanced endoplasmic reticulum stress, oxidative stress, and apoptosis that underlie neutropenia and neutrophil dysfunction. Neutrophil dysfunction may be secondary to defective chemotaxis. Glycogen storage disease type 1b leads to metabolic derangements and hepatic glycogen accumulation, fasting hypoglycemia, hyperuricemia, susceptibility to infections, and colitis [15, 22]. The marrow is often hypercellular with an ample number of neutrophils without any signs of maturation arrest [1]. Neutropenia and/or neutrophil dysfunction predisposes patients to frequent infections and inflammatory bowel disease, and is treated by G-CSF [11].

In addition to the aforementioned syndromes, there are several other distinct congenital syndromes including Shwachman-Diamond syndrome, dyskeratosis congenita, reticular dysgenesis, Pearson syndrome, Griscelli syndrome type II, warts, hypogammaglobulinemia, infections, and myelokatexis (WHIM) syndrome that present with neutropenia and a variety of other symptoms and signs.

II. Acquired Neutropenia

1. Immune Neutropenia

Immune neutropenia is the clinical entity caused by alloimmune or autoimmune antibodies directed against neutrophil specific glycoprotein antigens. Alloimmune neutropenia, also known as alloimmune neonatal neutropenia is the disease of the fetus or newborn caused by maternal sanitization to fetal antigens from paternal source. Any fetomaternal blood contact through transfusion, or hemorrhage leads to perception of fetal antigens by the mother's immune system as non-self, and results in production of allo-reactive IgG antibodies in maternal blood that crosses the placenta into the fetal circulation. Maternal antibodies are directed against neutrophil specific antigens NA1 and NA2 which are located on the FcγRIII receptor of fetal/newborn neutrophils. Affected newborns develop transient neutropenia that will ultimately recover after 11 weeks postpartum and generally, infectious complications are not common [4]. G-CSF can be administered when required.

Autoimmune neutropenia (AIN) is divided into primary and secondary forms. Primary AIN in adults is often a chronic disease with higher prevalence in females [20]; however, it is more common in early childhood than in adults. Children suffering from primary AIN develop mild to moderate infections and are less likely to have serious infections. Nevertheless, G-CSF along with antibiotics is warranted in recurrent or severe infectious complications [4].

Secondary AIN in adults manifest as part of systemic autoimmune disorders, malignancies, reaction to certain medications or infections such as HIV and hepatitis viruses. Just like red blood cells and platelets neutrophils have their own specific antigens, which are expressed on plasma membrane glycoprotiens. FcɤRIII (CD16) and 58-64kDa (CD177) are two different glycoproteins that the NA and NB neutrophilic antigens are expressed on them respectively. As a result of immune dysregulation in autoimmune neutropenia, neutrophilic glycoproteins are perceived as non-self or tolerances against these receptor-glycoproteins are distorted. Subsequently, IgG anti-neutrophilic antibodies will appear in the patient's blood. As previously stated, granulocyte immunofluorescence test (GIFT), granulocyte indirect immunofluorescence test (GIIFT), granulocyte agglutination test (GAT), enzyme linked immunoassays (ELISA) and monoclonal antibody-specific immobilization of granulocyte antigens (MAIGA) are just some of the methods that may detect anti-neutrophilic antibody. However, GAT and GIFT are more the test more commonly used [4, 20]. In general, testing for anti-neutrophil antibodies are less widely used in the light of specific challenges such as difficulty of interpretation, abundance of neutrophil receptors and its related false negative results and finally fragility of neutrophils [4]. Most of current understanding about mechanisms of neutrophil destruction in autoimmune neutropenia stems from in vitro observations. Agglutination is the major form of neutrophil response to antineutrophil antibodies. Complement mediated neutrophil agglutination in the presence of antineutrophil antibodies is another proposed mechanism. There is large body of evidence that activated complement can cause neutrophil aggregation and adherence to endothelial cells [16]. Each mechanism separately or in combination may lead to neutrophil apoptosis and clinically related neutropenia which in return lead to infectious syndromes. The most common forms of adult secondary AIN are discussed here.

Autoimmune Neutropenia in Felty's Syndrome

Classically, Felty's syndrome (FS) is characterized by a triad of rheumatoid arthritis (RA), neutropenia and splenomegaly. However, the latter is not required to establish the clinical diagnosis of FS. FS is an uncommon clinical entity, and the lifetime risk of developing FS in a patient with RA is 1-3% [16]. There is evidence that anti-neutrophilic antibody and immune complex adhering to neutrophils cause destruction and peripheral margination of neutrophils [20]. FS typically occurs in patients with longstanding RA and end-organ involvement of RA, including pulmonary fibrosis, vasculitis, rheumatoid nodules and splenomegaly. Emergence of FS may increase morbidity due to infectious complications and in very rare cases patients may succumb to overwhelming sepsis [4]. From a laboratory standpoint, FS patients have high levels of rheumatoid factor (RF), circulating immune complexes, and hypergammaglobulinemia. Anti-neutrophilic antibody is positive in most FS patients and 90% of patients are positive for HLA-DR4. These patients may have an elevated number of circulatory and bone marrow large granular lymphocytes (LGL) [16]. Demonstrating the characteristic immunophenotype of CD3+, CD8+, CD16+ and CD57+ and finding a clonal T cell receptor (TCR) gene rearrangement is diagnostic [4]. Proper antibiotic therapy with or without G-CSF is a common practice to manage neutropenic episodes in FS patient. G-CSF increases the production and release of mature neutrophils into circulation, and causes demarginalization of the neutrophils. G-CSF may also increase clearance of significant amount of anti-neutrophil antibodies from serum, and decrease neutrophil apoptosis. Down regulation of neutrophil membrane antigen expression by G-CSF results in reduced activity of autoantibodies [16].

Autoimmune Neutropenia in Systemic Lupus Erythematosus

Neutropenia is a common finding in patients with active SLE, and has been reported in approximately half (50-60%) of the SLE patients. Neutropenia secondary to SLE increases risk of infection. Bacterial infections occur in 80% of these patients which makes bacterial infection the second cause of death after cardiovascular complications [16]. There is growing evidence that Fas-mediated apoptosis of mature neutrophils is a major contributing factor in SLE-associated neutropenia, while there are other mechanisms including marrow hypoplasia and Fas-mediated apoptosis of CD34+ hematopoietic progenitor cells that contribute in neutropenia as well [4, 20]. It has been shown that in patient with SLE serum levels of tumor necrosis factor-related apoptosis-inducing ligand (TRAIL) were inversely proportional to blood neutrophil counts [16]. Neutropenia is SLE has been hypothesized to be pathologically related to the presence of anti-SSA (Ro) and anti-SSB (La) antibodies [4]. The main treatment of AIN in SLE is proper control of underlying disorder, G-CSF and antibiotics as needed.

Autoimmune Neutropenia due to Malignancy

Convincing data supports the fact that certain malignancies can cause AIN. For instance, AIN is a common finding in hairy cell leukemia patients, while in chronic lymphocytic leukemia the incidents is much lower (<1-2%) [20, 31]. Reports suggest that Hodgkin's lymphoma [32] and even Wilms tumor can also be associated with AIN [33].

Autoimmune Neutropenia due to Infections

Viral infections such as HIV are associated with secondary AIN in adults. Certain other infective agents like parvovirus B19, helicobacter pylori, Epstein-Barr Virus, and mycoplasma pneumoniae have also been reported to contribute to AIN [20, 33].

In addition to the aforementioned mechanisms, certain medications can also cause AIN which is described in the following section.

2. Drug-Induced Neutropenia

Drug-induced neutropenia is an adverse reaction of various medications and may increase infectious complications with a mortality of 2.5-10% [15]. This form of neutropenia is more common in women and elderly [34] and presence of renal failure, bacteremia and shock at the time of diagnosis has higher mortality rate [5]. Drug induced neutropenia may be caused by different immune mechanisms. Immune-mediated can be rapid in onset (e.g. penicillin), complement-mediated (e.g. propylthiouracil), acceleration of apoptosis (e.g. clozapine), dose dependent inhibition of granulopoiesis (e.g. carbamazepine), direct toxic effects on myeloid precursor (e.g. busulfan, methimazole) [34, 35]. Management of drug-induced neutropenia includes discontinuation of offending or presumed to be offending medications, good supportive care, proper antibiotic therapy and administration of G-CSF as required. Table 5 shows the list of medications that can cause neutropenia.

Table 5. Drugs associated with neutropenia (modified from Wintrobe's Clinical Hematology [36])

1. Analgesics/anti-inflammatory agents

- indomethacin
- ibuprofen
- aspirin
- mesalazine
- aminopyrine
- phenylbutazone
- barbiturates

2. Antipsychotics and antidepressants

- phenothiazines
- clozapine
- risperidone
- imipramine
- desipramine
- haloperidol

3. Anticonvulsants

- valproic acid
- carbamazepine
- phenytoin
- ethosuximide
- mesantoin

4. Antithyroid drugs

- thiouracil
- propylthiouracil
- carbimazole
- methimazole
- thiocyanate

5. Antihistaminics

- cimetidine
- ranitidine
- brompheniramine
- methapheniline

6. Antimicrobials

- penicillins
- cephalosporins
- chloramphenicol
- gentamicin
- metronidazole
- rifampin
- isoniazid
- pyrimethamine
- levamisole
- sulfonamides

- dapsone
- chloroquine
- acyclovir
- zidovudine
- ciprofloxacin

7. Cardiovascular drugs
- procainamide
- captopril
- propanolol
- hydralazine
- methyldopa
- nifedipine
- ticlopidine
- quinidine

8. Chemotherapy
- melphalan
- busulfan
- methotrexate
- carboplatin
- cisplatin
- cis-diammine-dichloroplatinum
- paclitaxel
- doxorubicin
- cyclophosphamide
- tetoposide
- venorelbine
- tyrosine kinase inhibitors [37]

9. Heavy metals
- gold compounds
- arsenic compounds
- mercury compounds

10. Miscellaneous drugs
- iv immunoglobulin
- allopurinol
- colchicine
- tamoxifen
- retinoic acid
- ethanol
- thiazide diuretics
- levodopa

3. Infection- Induced Neutropenia

The fact that neutropenia follows infections is straightforward and obviously explained as impaired defense against invasive pathogens. The reverse of above is also possible. There are certain microorganisms that can negatively affect neutrophils and lead to clinically significant neutropenia.

Parvovirus B19, HIV, helicobacter pylori, EBV, and mycoplasma are just some of the common organisms that may cause AIN [20, 33]. Helicobacter pylori and mycobacterium tuberculosis induced neutropenia secondary to splenomegaly have also been reported [38, 39]. Brucella melitensis, Yersinia enterocolitica, Chlamydia trachomatis, Listeria monocytogenes, parasites including Plasmodium falciparum, Toxoplasma gondii, Strongyloides ratii, fungi such as Aspergillus fumigatus and Candida albicans and viruses like cytomegalovirus, human herpesvirus-6 and influenza viruses have been reported as the etiology of neutropenia on rare occasions [40, 41, 42, 43]. Treatment includes proper antibiotic therapy in conjunction with G-CSF if indicated. In the event no treatment is available for the pathogen, supportive treatment will remain as the only option.

4. Hypersplenism

The basic pathology in hypersplenism that leads to neutropenia is the entrapment and subsequent destruction of neutrophils in the spleen. Hypersplenism may result from liver cirrhosis with portal hypertension, lymphoma, sarcoidosis, or Felty's syndrome [44]. The bone marrow cellularity is often increased with normal maturation sequence; however the survival of neutrophils is shortened.

5. Aplastic Anemia

Apastic anemia is characterized by incapacitated bone marrow to generate all tree blood cells lines with varying severity. The etiology of aplastic anemia could be viral infection, medications, chemicals or immune mechanisms [45]. No matter what the cause is, affected patients have low number of neutrophils which leads to susceptibility to infections. Management includes application of immunosuppressive or hematopoietic stem cell transplantation (HSCT).

6. Bone Marrow Replacement

Neutropenia and/or other cytopenias could be caused by bone marrow replacement by fibrotic tisse in myelofibrosis, metastatic cancerous cells originating from lung, prostate, stomach, and skin (such as malignant melanoma) [1]. Management includes appropriate supportive care and treatment of primary cause.

7. Vitamin B12/Folate and Copper Deficiency

Role of vitamin B_{12} and folate in the metabolism of DNA and cell maturation is well established. Patients with vitamin B_{12} or folate deficiency may develop neutropenia or pancytopenia due to dyssynchronous nuclear and cytoplasmic maturation. The bone marrow is hypercellular. Myeloid cells suffer a high degree of intramedullary death due to the effect of vitamin B_{12} or folate deficiency on nuclear replication [1]. Data indicates that an early clinical sign of copper deficiency is a reduction in the number of neutrophils [46]. The exact mechanism for copper-deficient neutropenia is not clear, although factors such as gastric resection, unsupplemented total parenteral nutrition, high levels of zinc intake, or general malnutrition are known to cause depleted body copper stores [46].

8. Irradiation

Ionization radiation may interact directly with intracellular targets or may interact with other molecules such as H_2O to produce free radicals that in turn involves DNA, plasma membrane and other cellular structures. The phenomenon of radiation ionization is universal and neutrophils are not exception to this general rule. Exposure to ionizing radiation may be accidental or therapeutic. The extent of neutrophil injury will vary based on the amount and length of exposure, [47]. Concurrent administration of chemotherapy and radiotherapy may even increase the chance of myelosuppression including neutropenia. Management includes aggressive supportive care consists of antibiotics, blood products, and fluids as well as administration of G-CSF as soon as possible after exposure [47]. However use of G-CSF while radiotherapy is ongoing might lead to more severe neutropenia in view of the fact that it will stimulate the production of more neutrophils which could be damaged by the on-going radiotherapy. Thus the use of G-CSF should be avoided during radiotherapy.

9. Acquired Disorders of Myeloid Stem Cells

Hematologic malignancies can lead to bone marrow compromise and cause neutropenia. Common causes include but are not limited to acute myelogenous leukemia, myelodysplastic syndrome, and multiple myeloma [1,]. Another challenge would be the emergence of neutropenia while treating these malignancies with chemotherapy. Management includes eradicating the actual cause, proper antibiotic therapy and G-CSF.

10. Granulomatous Diseases and Neutropenia

Granulomatous diseases such as tuberculosis and rheumatologic diseases like rheumatoid arthritis causing neutropenia have already been discussed. Certain other granulomatous diseases for instance sarcoidosis can cause neutropenia [48]. The association of Crohn's disease with cyclic neutropenia [49] and autoimmune neutropenia has been reported as well [50].

Management

Depending on its etiology, severity, duration and the estimated risk, the management of neutropenia is multifaceted and can be challenging. In situations where the etiology of neutropenia is drug-related, the offending agents must be stopped promptly and supportive care should be initiated as soon as possible. If the cause is related to nutritional deficiency, proper replacement is warranted. Preventive measures like proper and frequent hand washing, avoiding crowded areas, practicing good oral hygiene, careful skin care, and consuming proper diet can help to decrease chance of getting infected. Central lines and intravenous catheters should be properly monitored.

The important therapeutic goal in treating neutropenic patients is the reconstitution of adequate neutrophil counts by G-CSF or the treatment of the underling cause. G-CSF is a polypeptide growth factor which is produced by bone marrow cells, endothelial cells, macrophages and fibroblasts [16]. G-CSF increases neutrophil counts by enhancing neutrophil production, inducing neutrophil demarginalization and subsequent clearance of neutrophils, reduction of neutrophil apoptosis and down regulating neutrophil membrane antigen expression through JAK/STAT signaling pathway. Different preparations of G-CSF have been produced by recombinant technology and introduced for clinical use. Filgrastim is very similar to endogenous G-CSF with the exception of having an added N-terminal methionine. Pegfilgrastim has polyethylene glycol bound to the N-terminal methionine, and Lenograstim is a glycosylated preparation of G-CSF [51]. Despite slight differences in chemical structure, all of them interact with G-CSF receptor and initiate their effects similarly. Some of G-CSF side effects include but are not limited to bone pain, headache, fatigue, nausea, fever, thrombocytopenia, osteoporosis and injection site reactions [52]. Another growth factor called Sargarmostin [53], a granulocyte monocyte- colony stimulating factor (GM-CSF), is also used in neutropenic settings, especially when the patient is suffering from concomitant monocytopenia.

Antibiotics are used both for prophylaxis and treatment of infectious syndromes as neutropenic patients are prone to become infected in the light of decreased neutrophil counts. For the management of bacterial infections proper antibiotics should be administered after appropriate sensitivity testing, unless in overwhelming infections which empirical regimens are life-saving and are accepted as standard of care. The administration of antibiotics in inpatient or outpatient settings should be weighed according to the stability of the patient and severity of infection status. Bacterial infections are becoming more and more resistant to current antibiotics, and thus certain strategies should be applied in order to prevent bacterial resistance. Choosing antibiotics is judged based upon the etiologic agents and available practice guidelines introduced by professional organizations such as Infectious diseases Society of America (IDSA) can be helpful.

Fungal infections usually occur in long standing neutropenias such as bone marrow recipients with delayed engraftment. Candida, aspergillus species, and zygomycosis are among commonly fungal agents implicated in neutropenic patients. There is more detailed information regarding fungal infections of neutropenic patients and their treatments in the literature [40, 54, 55, 56, 57].

Conclusion

Neutropenia can be caused by a wide range of congenital and acquired disorders. Realtime elucidation of neutropenic causes is essential to avoid huge numbers of morbidities and mortalities in clinical settings. The evaluation of neutropenic patients starts with obtaining a thorough medical history and performing a skillful physical exam followed by proper laboratory assessment; even though critical patient might not warrant this sequence in the light of life-threatening conditions. The application of sophisticated medical technology, the introduction of G-CSF and worthwhile antimicrobial agents have opened new horizons for the fast and reliable recovery of neutropenic patients.

References

[1] Boxer L, Dale DC (2002). Neutropenia: Causes and Consequences. *Semin Hematol* 39(2):75-81.

[2] Hsieh MM, Everhart JE, Byrd-Holt DD and et al. (2007). Prevalence of Neutropenia in the U.S. Population: Age, Sex, Smoking Status, and Ethnic Differences. *Ann Intern Med.* 146(7):486-492.

[3] Chindaprasirt J, Wanitpongpun C, Limpawattana P, Thepsuthammarat K, Sripakdee W, Wirasorn K, Sookprasert A (2013). Mortality, Length of Stay, and Cost Associated with Hospitalized Adult Cancer Patients with Febrile Neutropenia. *Asian Pacific J Cancer Prev,* 14 (2), 1115-1119.

[4] Berliner N, Horzwitz M, Loughran TP Jr (2004). Congenital and Acquired Neutropenia. *Hematology* 63-79.

[5] Vanderberghe P and Beel K (2011). Severe congenital neutropenia, a genetically heterogeneous disease group with an increased risk of AML/MDS. *Pediatric Reports* 3(s2):e9.

[6] Fernandez BA, Green JS, Bursey F and et al. (2012). Adult siblings with homozygous G6PC3 mutations expand our understanding of the severe congenital neutropenia type 4 (SCN4) phenotype. BMC Medical Genetics 13:111.

[7] Gahl WA, Huizing M. Hermansky-Pudlak Syndrome. 2000 Jul 24 [Updated 2013 Feb 28]. In: Pagon RA, Adam MP, Bird TD, et al., editors. GeneReviews™ [Internet]. Seattle (WA): University of Washington, Seattle; 1993-2013. Available from: http://www.ncbi.nlm.nih.gov/books/NBK1287/.

[8] Dale CD, Bolyark AA, Aprikyan A (2002). Cyclic neutropenia. *Semin Hematol* 39(2):89-94.

[9] Aprikyan AA, Liles WC, Park JR and et al. (2000). Myelokathexis, a congenital disorder of severe neutropenia characterized by accelerated apoptosis and defective expression of bcl-x in neutrophil precursors. *Blood* 95(1):320-327.

[10] Chou JY, Sik Jun H, Mansfield BC (2010). Neutropenia in type Ib glycogen storage disease. *Curr Opin Hematol.* 17(1): 36–42.

[11] Kim SY, Jun HS, Mead PA, Mansfield BC, Chou JY (2008). Neutrophil stress and apoptosis underlie myeloid dysfunction in glycogen storage disease type Ib. *Blood.* 15;111(12):5704-11.

[12] Rommens JM, Durie PR. *Shwachman-Diamond Syndrome.* 2008 Jul 17. In: Pagon RA, Adam MP, Bird TD, et al., editors. GeneReviews™ [Internet]. Seattle (WA): University of Washington, Seattle; 1993-2013. Available from: http://www.ncbi.nlm.nih.gov/books/NBK1756/.

[13] Hsieh MW, Tisdale JF, Rodger GP et al. (2010). Neutrophil Counts in African Americans: Lowering the Target Cutoff to Initiate or Resume Chemotherapy? *J Clin Oncol.* 28(10): 1633-1637.

[14] van Staa TP, Boulton F, Cooper C and et al. (2003). Neutropenia and Agranulocytosis in England and Wales: Incidence and Risk Factors. American Journal of Hematology 72(4):248–254.

[15] Boxer LA (2012). How to Approach Neutropenia. *Hematology*. 174-182.

[16] Newman KA, Akhtari M (2011). Management of autoimmune neutropenia in Felty's syndrome and systemic lupus erythematosus. *Autoimmunity Reviews* 10(7):432–437.

[17] Rolston KV (2009). Bacterial infection in neutropenic cancer patients: an overview. *Iranian Journal of Clinical Infectious Diseases* 4(2):115-122.

[18] Rolston KV (2004). Management of infections in the neutropenic patient. *Annu. Rev. Med.* 55:519–526.

[19] Tfayli A, Gadde L, Shamseddin Ali (2010). Pseudoneutropenia from EDTA Leukoagglutination. *Middle East Journal of Cancer* 1(4): 189-190.

[20] Akhtari M, Curtis B, Waller EK (2009). Autoimmune neutropenia in adults. *Autoimmunity Reviews* 9(1): 62–66.

[21] Klein C (2009). Congenital neutropenia. *Hematology* 344-350.

[22] Donadieu J, Fenneteau O, Beaupain B et al. (2011). Congenital Neutropenia: diagnosis, molecular basis and patient management. *Orphanet Journal of Rare Diseases* 6:26.

[23] Wenham M, Grieve S, Cummins M and et al. (2010). Two patients with Hermansky Pudlak syndrome type 2 and novel mutation in AP3B1. *Haematologica* 95(2) 333-337.

[24] Dotta, L., Parolini, S., Prandini, A., Tabellini, G., Antolini, M., Kingsmore, S. F., & Badolato, R. (2013). Clinical, laboratory and molecular signs of immunodeficiency in patients with partial oculo-cutaneous albinism. *Orphanet Journal of Rare Diseases*, *8*, 168. doi:10.1186/1750-1172-8-168

[25] Fantinato GT, Cestari Sda C, Afonso JP, Sousa LS, Enokihara MMSS. Você conhece esta síndrome? (2011) Síndrome de Chediak-Higashi. *An Bras Dermatol.* 86(5):1029-38.

[26] de Azambuja AP, do Nascimento B and et all (2011). Four cases of Chédiak-Higashi syndrome. *Rev Bras Hematol Hemoter* 33(4):315-322.

[27] de Lonlay and Schlemmer D (2005). *Barth Syndrome. Orphanet Encyclopedia.*https://www.orpha.net/data/patho/GB/uk-BarthSyndrome.pdf.

[28] Clarke et al. (2013): Barth syndrome. *Orphanet Journal of Rare Diseases* 8:23.

[29] Falk MJ, Wang H, Traboulsi EI. Cohen Syndrome. 2006 Aug 29 [Updated 2011 Mar 10]. In: Pagon RA, Adam MP, Bird TD, et al., editors. GeneReviews™ [Internet]. Seattle (WA): University of Washington, Seattle; 1993-2013. Available from: http://www.ncbi.nlm.nih.gov/books/NBK1482/.

[30] Kim SY, Jun HS, Mead PA, Mansfield BC, Chou JY (2008). Neutrophil stress and apoptosis underlie myeloid dysfunction in glycogen storage disease type Ib. *Blood.* 15;111(12):5704-11.

[31] Hodgson K, Ferrer G, Montserrat E, Moreno C (2011). Chronic lymphocytic leukemia and autoimmunity: a systematic review. *Haematologica.* 96(5):752-761.

[32] Lechner K, Chen YA (2010). Paraneoplastic autoimmune cytopenias in Hodgkin lymphoma. *Leuk Lymphoma.* 51(3):469-474.

[33] Capsoni F, Sarzi-Puttini P, Zanella A (2005). Primary and secondary autoimmune neutropenia. *Arthritis Res Ther.* 7(5):208-214.

[34] Bhatt V, Saleem A (2004). Review: Drug-Induced Neutropenia – Pathophysiology, Clinical Features, and Management. *Annals of Clinical & Laboratory Science* 34(2)131- 137.

[35] Mintzer DM, Billet SN, Chmielewski L (2009). Drug-induced hematologic syndromes. *Adv Hematol.* 495863. doi: 10.1155/2009/495863.

[36] Watts RG (2013). Neutropenia. In: *Wintrobe's Clinical Hematology,* 13th Ed, (Lee GR, Foerster J, Lukens J, Eds). Baltimore, Williams and Wilkins, pp 1279-1290.

[37] Barber NA, Afzal W, Akhtari M (2011). Hematologic toxicities of small molecule tyrosine kinase inhibors. *Targ Oncol* 6(4):203- 215.

[38] Papadaki HA, Pontikoglou C, Eliopoulus DG and et al. (2006). Helicobacter pylori Infection is Probably the Cause of Chronic Idiopathic Neutropenia (CIN)- Associated Splenomegaly. *America Journal of Hematology* 81(2):142-144.

[39] Azzam, N. A. (2013). Splenic tuberculosis presenting as fever of unknown origin with severe neutropenia. *Annals of Clinical Microbiology and Antimicrobials*, *12*, 13. doi:10.1186/1476-0711-12-13

[40] Donowitz GR, Maki DG, Crnich CJ and et al. (2001). Infections in the Neutropenic Patient–New Views of an Old Problem. *Hematology* 113-139.

[41] Sari R, Buyukberber N, Sevinc A, Bayindir Y, Buyukberber S. (2002). Brucellosis in the etiology of febrile neutropenia: case report. J Chemother. 14(1): 88-91.

[42] Citak EC and Arman D (2011). *Brucella melitensis: a are cause of febrile neutropenia.* 28(1): 83-85..

[43] Sheen JM, Kuo HC, Yu HR, and et al. (2009). Prolonged acquired neutropenia in children. *Pediatr Blood Cancer.* 15;53(7):1284-1288.

[44] 92 Elmakii E (2012). Hypersplenism: Review article. *Journal of Biology, Agriculture and Healthcare.* 2(10): 89-99.

[45] Mavroudi I, Papadaki HA (2012). Genetic associations in acquired immune-mediated bone marrow failure syndromes: insights in aplastic anemia and chronic idiopathic neutropenia. *Clin Dev Immunol.* 123789. doi: 10.1155/2012/123789.

[46] Jabbour N, DiGiuseppe JA, Usmani S, Tannenbaum S (2010). Copper deficiency as a cause of reversible anemia and neutropenia. *Conn Med* 74(5):261-263

[47] Dainiak N, Waselenko JK, Armitage JO, MacVittie TJ, Farese AM (2003). The hematologist and radiation casualties. *Hematology Am Soc Hematol Educ Program.* 473-496.

[48] Chaudhary P, Gopaluni S, Sanyal S, Shah C (2010). Atypical sarcoidosis masquerading as neutropenia. *Sarcoidosis vasculitis and diffuse lung diseases* 27(2); 160-163.

[49] Lamport RD, Katz S, Eskreis D (1992). Crohn's disease associated with cyclic neutropenia. *Am J Gastroenterol.* 87(11):1638-1642.

[50] Stevens C, Peppercorn MA, Grand RJ (1991). Crohn's diease associated with autoimmune neutropenia. *J Clin Gastroenterol.* 13(3):328-30.

[51] Kouroukis CT, Chia S, Verma S and et al. (2008). Canadian supportive care recommendations for the management of neutropenia in patients with cancer. *Current Oncology* 15(1):9-23.

[52] Cottle TE, Fier CJ, Donadieu J, Kinsey SE (2002). Risk and Benefit of Treatment of Severe Chronic Neutropenia with Granulocyte Colony-Stimulating Factor. *Semin Hematol* 39(2):134-140.

[53] Gabay M, Tanzi M (2009). Guideline for the Management of Febrile Neutropenia. *Pharmacy Practice Reviews* 8-17.

[54] Aguilar-Guisado M, Martín-Peña A, Espigado I, Ruiz Pérez de Pipaon M, Falantes J, de la Cruz F, and Cisneros JM (2012). Universal antifungal therapy is not needed in persistent febrile neutropenia: a tailored diagnostic and therapeutic approach. *Haematologica* 97(3): 464-471.

[55] Shalhoub, S., Wang, L., Ching, A., Husain, S., & Rotstein, C. (2014). Micafungin compared with caspofungin for the treatment of febrile episodes in neutropenic patients with hematological malignancies: A retrospective study. *The Canadian Journal of Infectious Diseases & Medical Microbiology*, *25*(6), 299–304.

[56] Gedik, H., Şimşek, F., Yıldırmak, T., Kantürk, A., Arıca, D., Aydın, D., … Yokuş, O. (2014). Primary or secondary antifungal prophylaxis in patients with hematological maligancies: efficacy and damage. *Therapeutics and Clinical Risk Management*, *10*, 305–312.

[57] Kim, S.-J., Cheong, J.-W., Min, Y. H., Choi, Y. J., and et al. (2014). Success Rate and Risk Factors for Failure of Empirical Antifungal Therapy with Itraconazole in Patients with Hematological Malignancies: A Multicenter, Prospective, Open-Label, Observational Study in Korea. *Journal of Korean Medical Science*, *29*(1), 61–68.

In: Neutropenia
Editors: M. Akhtari et al.
ISBN: 978-1-63482-105-6

Chapter 2

Drug-Induced Neutropenia

Adrienne N. Nedved[1] *and Mojtaba Akhtari*[2]
[1]Department of Pharmacy, Mayo Clinic Hospital, Rochester, MN, US
[2]Jane Anne Nohl Division of Hematology and Center for the Study of Blood Diseases, University of Southern California (USC)/ Norris Cancer Center, USC University Hospital, Keck Medical Center of USC, Los Angeles, CA, US

Introduction

While various definitions and degrees of neutropenia exist, neutropenia as described throughout this book is generally defined as an absolute neutrophil count (ANC) of <500/microL or <0.5 x 10^9/L. [1-4] Neutropenia can be divided into two broad classifications: acquired or intrinsic, with acquired neutropenia being more common. Acquired neutropenia that develops secondary to use of a drug is further classified as drug-induced neutropenia. Drug-induced neutropenia has been documented with a number of medications, both cytotoxic and non-cytotoxic drugs, but is most commonly related to antineoplastic medications. Drug-induced neutropenia caused by non-cytotoxic agents, the focus of this chapter, is also known as drug-induced agranulocytosis (DIAG) and can be life-threatening [5-7]. Similarly, drug-induced agranulocytosis is defined as an ANC <500/microL; however, most cases present with an ANC <100/microL [5, 8].

Epidemiology and Risk Factors

Drug-induced agranulocytosis is a rare condition with variable pathophysiology that is based on differences in pharmacological, toxic, and biochemical properties not only between the various drug classes, but also among the specific agents within those classes [6]. Because of the diversity in drug properties responsible for potentially causing agranulocytosis and the rarity of the condition, there is limited data available regarding the topic. However, one international multi-center study conducted in Europe and Israel assessed idiopathic severe neutropenia cases in a general population and found that drugs were responsible for causing approximately 62% of the reported cases, which equated to 3.4 cases per million per year [9-10]. In comparison to the rates of DIAG in Europe and Israel, the United States had a separate study that reported drug-induced agranulocytosis incidence rates between 2.4 to 15.4 per million per year [11]. Of note, additional European studies report incidence rates for drug-induced agranulocytosis ranging from 1.6 to 9.2 per million [12-17].

Only about 10% of reported cases of drug-induced agranulocytosis occurred in the pediatric and young adult populations, while more than half of the reported cases occurred in adults over the age of sixty [16-18]. A possible cause for the increased incidence of drug-induced agranulocytosis in elderly patients is that they tend to have been exposed to a significantly increased number of drugs than the pediatric and young adult patients [12]. Additionally, the rate of drug-induced agranulocytosis has been reported twice as frequently in females compared to males [18-19]. One theory to explain this is that there is an increased use of pertinent drugs in females due to longer life expectancy compared with males, which may bias the data [18-19].

Additional risk factors for drug-induced agranulocytosis not due to cytotoxic chemotherapy include: renal insufficiency, genetic predisposition, autoimmune disease, and combinations of paticular drugs (Table 1) [8, 10]. Renal insufficiency may increase the risk of developing drug-induced agranulocytosis with certain drugs, specifically when drugs that are cleared through the renal system are used in combination, such as captopril and probenecid [20]. Because of a potential decrease in clearance of these drugs, there is an increased risk for drug accumulation. Several studies suggest that an underlying autoimmune disorder such as rheumatoid arthritis, [8, 21-22] or presence of particular histocompatibility antigens such as HLA-B27 and HLA-B38 may predispose patients to an increased risk for developing drug-induced agranulocytosis with drugs such as methimazole and clozapine [8, 21, 23-24].

Conversely, one study reported that the presence of HLA-B35 may actually protect patients from developing drug-induced agranulocytosis related to the use of clozapine [25].

Table 1. Risk Factors for Developing Drug-Induced Agranulocytosis [8, 10, 12, 16-25, 31]

Elderly Age
Female Gender
Renal Impairment
Genetics (presence of certain histocompatibility antigens)
Autoimmune Disorders

Drugs Associated with Drug-Induced Neutropenia

Many drug classes have been associated with drug-induced agranulocytosis; however, incidence rates are usually based upon case reports and tend to be very low for most of the drugs involved. Table 2 provides a list of the drugs most commonly identified with non-cytotoxic drug-induced agranulocytosis [8-9, 12-14, 18, 22, 26-38]. Drug classes most commonly implicated with drug-induced agranulocytosis include anti-infectives, antipsychotics, antiepileptics, nonsteroidal anti-inflammatory drugs, antithyroid drugs, and certain cardiovascular medications [8-9, 12-14, 18, 22, 26-38].

Table 2. Drugs Related to Drug-Induced Agranulocytosis [8-9, 12-14, 18, 22, 26-38]

Drug Class	Specific Agents
Analgesics and Nonsteroidal Anti-inflammatory Drugs:	Acetasalicylic acid; Acetaminophen; Diclofenac; Fenoprofen Ibuprofen; Indomethacin; Naproxen; Piroxicam; Sulindac
Antidepressants/ Antianxiety Agents:	Amoxapine; Fluoxetine; Imipramine; Meprobamate

Table 2. (Continued)

Drug Class	Specific Agents
Antipsychotics:	Clozapine; Haloperidol; Olanzapine; Phenothiazines; Risperidone; Thioridazine; Ziprasidone
Antiepileptics:	Carbamazepine; Ethosuximide; Lamotrigine; Phenytoin; Valproic acid
Antithyroid drugs:	Methimazole; Propylthiouracil
Antihistamines:	Brompheniramine; Chlorpheniramine; Imipramine
Anti-infectives:	Abacavir; Atovaquone; Beta-Lactams: *Ampicillin, Amoxicillin-clavulanic acid, Cloxacillin, Nafcillin, Oxacillin, Penicillin, Piperacillin, Ticarcillin;* Cephalosporins: *Cefepime, Cefotaxime, Ceftriaxone, Cefuroxime, Cephalexin;* Chloroquine; Ciprofloxacin; Clarithromycin; Clindamycin; Dapsone; Ethambutol; Flucytosine; Ganciclovir; Gentamicin; Griseofulvin; Imipenem-cilastatin; Indinavir; Isoniazid; Linezolid; Metronidazole; Minocycline; Nitrofurantoin; Quinine; Rifampicin; Streptomycin; Sulfamethoxazole-Trimethoprim; Terbinafine; Tetracycline; Tinidazole; Valganciclovir; Vancomycin; Zidovudine
Benzodiazepines:	Chlordiazepoxide; Diazepam
Cardiovascular Drugs:	Amiodarone; Captopril; Clopidogrel; Dipyridamole; Digoxin; Furosemide; Hydralazine; Lisinopril; Methyldopa; Metolazone; Nifedipine; Procainamide; Propafenone; Propranolol; Quinidine; Ramipril; Spironolactone; Thiazide diuretics; Ticlopidine
Gastrointestinal Drugs:	Histamine (H2) Antagonists: *Cimetidine, Famotidine, Ranitidine;* Mesalazine; Metoclopramide; Omeprazole
Miscellaneous Drugs:	Allopurinol; Chlorpropamide; Colchicine; Glucocorticoids; Hydroxychloroquine; Levodopa; Methazolamide; Sulfasalazine

Pathophysiology

While the pathophysiology behind drug-induced agranulocytosis is not fully understood, several pathophysiologic mechanisms have been suggested by past clinical observations and studies [8, 12, 30].

The most common proposed mechanisms can be classified as either an immune-mediated reaction or direct-toxicity from the medication [8, 12, 30, 59]. Sometimes a combination of those two pathophysiologic pathways has also been suggested when analyzing drug-induced agranulocytosis in patients [31].

Immune-mediated drug-induced agranulocytosis is thought to occur either following prolonged periods of exposure to the offending agent or through repeated intermittent exposures; however, this theory is still under investigation [12, 39]. The presence of antineutrophil antibodies has been established in drug-induced agranulocytosis caused by medications such as beta-lactam antibiotics, chlorpropramide, and antithyroid medications,. [8, 12, 40-45] It is hypothesized that these medications induce the production of the antineutrophil antibodies. The circulating antibodies then bind to target cells, and bind complement when exposed to one of the contributing medications [8, 12, 46].

Drug-induced agranulocytosis caused by direct-toxicity from the medication occurs through damage to the myeloid precursor cells [8, 12, 13]. When genetic polymorphisms are present in the metabolic pathways used to detoxify and eliminate medications, toxic metabolites and compounds may accumulate [8, 12, 47]. This can lead to damage of precursor cells and may cause cell death [8, 12, 13].

In addition, some medications such as cimetidine and quinidine have been shown to cause dose-dependent bone marrow suppression [31, 48-49]. Other pathways for direct toxicity damage from medication include direct neutrophil toxicity, such as that seen with sulfonamides [50] and increased rates of apoptosis with the use of clozapine [51].

Clinical Presentation and Diagnosis

Patients with drug-induced agranulocytosis typically present with sign and symptom onset of 7-14 days following initiation of therapy; however other references cite that some agents have been associated with extended periods of time to onset, ranging between 30-60 days [5, 13, 31]. Signs and symptoms may include sore throat, fever, infection, malaise, and sepsis [8, 18, 22, 30, 31, 52] with elderly patients at risk for presenting with more severe signs and symptoms [8, 53-54]. In contrast, less than one-fifth of patients may present without any symptoms initially [8, 55-56].

For patients suspected of drug-induced agranulocytosis, other causes of neutropenia should be excluded. Conditions to consider in the differential include: neutropenia secondary to infection, particularly due to severe sepsis, human immunodeficiency virus, or other viral syndromes; hypersplenism; autoimmune disorders, such as systemic lupus erythematosus; or neutropenia secondary to bone marrow failure from an underlying malignant condition, such as myelodisplastic syndrome, lymphoma, or leukemia [8, 22, 29, 31, 57-59]. Commonly, in order to rule out infiltrative marrow conditions such as malignancy, a bone marrow biopsy may be required [8, 12, 31]. With agranulocytosis, the bone marrow biopsy would demonstrate normo- to hypocellularity with normal erythroid lineage and megakaryocytes [8, 12, 22, 30, 53]. Myeloid precursor cells would be decreased or absent in the bone marrow, and mature neutrophils may be absent as well [8, 12, 22, 30, 53]. Laboratory tests, such as the granulocyte immunofluorescence test (GIFT) and the granulocyte agglutination test (GAT), also may be useful in assisting with diagnosis [59]. Both GIFT and GAT assess for the presence of antineutrophil cytoplasmic antibodies (ANCA), which have been found to be associated with drug-induced agranulocytosis [59-60].

Prognosis

Morbidity and mortality related to drug-induced agranulocytosis vary based on the causative agent, as well as the degree of neutropenia and the availability of antibiotic therapy. Mortality rates from case reports range from 0% to 23%; [13-14, 16, 21, 32, 61-63] however, a review of drug-induced agranulocytosis studies in Europe suggests a more recent overall mortality rate closer to 5% (range of 2.5 to 10%) [8, 12-13, 18]. This reduction from earlier reported overall mortality rates in Europe of 10-16% [8, 21, 30] is thought to be due to improvements in identifying and managing drug-induced agranulocytosis [8, 12-13, 18].

Management

The first step in managing drug-induced agranulocytosis is to identify potential causative agents [8, 12, 22, 30-31]. Once a likely causative agent has been identified, it should be discontinued immediately [8, 12, 22, 30-31]. This requires obtaining a thorough chronological medication history to identify agents that were started during the appropriate time frame [8, 12]. Bone marrow recovery following discontinuation of the offending agent(s) occurs in a median of 9 days, and ranges from two days to greater than two weeks [22, 31, 64]. Following discontinuation, the implicated drug should be documented as a contraindicated medication in the patient's medical record[64]. Other drugs that fall within the same chemical structure or drug class as the contraindicated drug should also be avoided whenever possible [31].

Cultures should be obtained and antibiotics initiated in patients who are febrile or show other signs of infection [8, 31, 64]. In particular, patients who have suspected sepsis should receive prompt, aggressive broad-spectrum antibiotic therapy [8, 22, 30, 53, 65-66]. Antibiotic therapy for the prevention of secondary infections is also recommended [8, 22, 30, 53]. Current IDSA guidelines for antimicrobial use in neutropenic patients with cancer recommend appropriate empiric antibiotic selection that includes coverage for *Pseudomonas aeruginosa* [64, 67]. Empiric antibiotic therapy should be continued at least until the absolute neutrophil count is greater than 500 cells/mm^3 or longer if clinically indicated [64, 67].

The use of hematopoietic growth factors in patients with drug-induced agranulocytosis has been assessed in a number of cohort studies, case-control studies, and systematic case reviews dating back to the 1990s. Andres et al. completed a systematic review of the existing data and concluded that the available evidence appears to support the use of hematopoietic growth factors in drug-induced agranulocytosis, especially in patients with one or more poor prognostic factors [64]. Poor prognostic factors include age greater than 65 years, severe agranulocytosis (absolute neutrophil count <100 cells/mm^3), severe concurrent infection, and pre-existing co-morbidities [12, 13, 21, 64, 68]. The available studies have demonstrated that hematopoietic growth factors appear to decrease the time to hematologic recovery, as well as the length of hospital stay and use of antibiotics [64]. While it is acknowledged that drug-induced agranulocytosis is not a U.S. Food and Drug Administration (FDA) labeled indication, Andres et al. have recommended to dose granulocyte colony-stimulating factors at 5μg/kg/day starting at the time of diagnosis [64]. In the studies, duration of hematopoietic growth factor administration was determined by time to hematologic recovery, which was defined as a rise in the neutrophil count to a specified level. The goal neutrophil count varied among studies; however, most studies continued hematopoietic growth factors until the absolute neutrophil count was above $1000/mm^3$ or $1500/mm^3$ [18, 64-66, 69-72].

Summary

Drug-induced agranulocytosis is a rare but potentially life-threatening condition that can occur following the administration of associated non-cytotoxic medications. Some of the most commonly reported classes of medications include antimicrobial agents, antithyroid medications, and antipsychotics. Patients who develop drug-induced agranulocytosis should discontinue the causative drug(s) immediately. Patients who are febrile or show signs of infection should be started on broad-spectrum antibiotics after obtaining appropriate cultures. The administration of hematopoietic growth factors may be considered, especially in patients with poor prognostic factors, to decrease time to hematologic recovery.

References

[1] Standardization of definitions and criteria of causality assessment of adverse drug reactions. Drug-induced cytopenia. *Int. J. Clin. Pharmcol. Ther. Toxicol.,* 1991;29:75-81.

[2] Palmblad JE, won dem Borne AE. Idiopathic, immune, infectious, and idiosyncratic neutropenias. *Semin. Hematol.,* 2002;39:113-120.

[3] Pizzo P. Management of fever in patients with cancer and treatment-induced neutropenia. *N. Engl. J. Med.,* 1993;328:1323-1332.

[4] Pisciotta AV. Drug-induced agranulocytosis. Peripheral destruction of polymorphonuclear leukocytes and their marrow precursors. *Transfus Med. Rev.,* 1990;4:226-237.

[5] Tesfa D, Keisu M, and Palmblad J. Idiosyncratic drug-induced agranulocytosis: Possible mechanisms and management. *Am. J. Hematol.,* 2009;84:428-434.

[6] Pisciotta AV. Drug-induced agranulocytosis. *Drugs.* 1976;15:132-143.

[7] Pisciotta AV. Drug-induced leukopenia and aplastic anemia. *Clin. Pharmacol. Ther.,* 1971;12:13-43.
[8] Andres E, Zimmer J, Affenberger, et al. Idiosyncratic drug-induced agranulocytosis: Update of an old disorder. *Eur. J. Intern. Med.,* 2006;17(8):529-535.
[9] Kaufman DW, Kelly JP, Jurgelon JM, et al. Drugs in the aetiology of agranulocytosis and aplastic anaemia. *Eur. J. Hematol.,* 1996;60:23-30.
[10] Young NS. Agranulocytosis. *JAMA.* 1994;271:935-938.
[11] Strom BL, Carson JL, Schinnar R, et al. Descriptive epidemiology of agranulocytosis. *Arch. Intern. Med.,* 1992;152:1475-1480.
[12] Andres E, Maloisel F. Idiosyncratic drug-induced agranulocytosis or acute neutropenia. *Curr. Opin. Hematol.,* 2008;15:15-21.
[13] Andersohn F, Konzen C, Garbe E. Systematic Review: Agranulocytosis induced by nonchemotherapy drugs. *Ann. Intern. Med.*, 2007;146:657-665.
[14] Van der Klauw MM, Goudsmit R, Halie MR, et al. A population-based case-cohort study of drug-associated agranulocytosis. *Arch. Intern. Med.,* 1999;159:369-374.
[15] Van Staa TP, Boulton F, Cooper C, et al. Neutropenia and agranylocytosis in England and Wales: incidence and risk factors. *Am. J. Hematol.,* 2003;72:248-254.
[16] Ibanez L, Vial X, Ballarin E, et al. Population-based drug-induced agranulocytosis. *Arch. Intern. Med.*, 2005;165:869-874.
[17] Theophile H, Begaud B, Martin K, et al. Incidence of agranulocytosis in Southwest France. *Eur. J. Epidemiol.,* 2004;19:563-565.
[18] Andres E, Maloisel F, Kurtz J, et al. Modern management of nonchemotherapy drug-induced agranulocytosis: a monocentric cohort study of 90 cases and review of the literature. *Eur. J. Intern. Med.,* 2002;13:324-328.
[19] Ma J, Alvir J, Lieberman J, et al. Clozapine-induced agranulocytosis. *N Engl. J. Med.,* 1993;329:162-167.
[20] Sinhvi S, Duchin K, Willard D, et al. Renal handling of captopril: effect of probenecid. *Clin. Pharmacol. Ther.,* 1982;32:182-189.
[21] Julia A, Olona M, Bueno J, et al. Drug-induced agranulocytosis: prognostic factors in a series of 168 patients. *Br. J. Haematol.*, 1991;79:366-371.
[22] Andres E, Kurtz J, Maloisel F. Non-chemotherapy drug-induced agranulocytosis: experience of the Strasbourg teaching hospital (1985-

2000) and review of the literature. *Clin. Lab. Haematol.,* 2002;24:99-106.

[23] Tamai H, Sudo T, Kimura A, et al. Association between the DRB108032 histocompatibility antigen and methimazole-induced agranulocytosis in Japanese patients with Graves' disease. *Ann. Intern. Med.,* 1996;124: 490-494.

[24] Hodinka L, Geher P, Meretey K, et al. Levamisole-induced neutropenia and agranulocytosis: association with HLA B27 leukocyte agglutinating and lymphocytotoxic antibodies. *Int. Arch. Allergy Appl. Immunol.,* 1981;65:460-464.

[25] Dettling M, Cascorbi I, Roots I, et al. Genetic determinants of clozapine-induced agranulocytosis: recent results of HLA subtyping in a non-Jewish Caucasian sample. *Arch. Gen. Psychiatry,* 2001;58:93-94.

[26] Heimpel H. Drug-induced agranulocytosis. *Medl. Toxicol.,* 1988;3:449-462.

[27] Paitel J, Stockemer V, Dorvaux V, et al. Acute drug-induced agranulocytosis. Clinical study of 30 patients: evolution of etiologies over 2 decades. *Rev. Med. Interne,* 1995;16:495-499.

[28] Vial T, Pofilet C, Pham E, et al. Acute drug-induced agranulocytosis: experience of the Regional Center of Pharmacovigilance of Lyon over 7 years. *Therapie,* 1996;51:508-515.

[29] Young N, Alter B. Agranulocytosis. Aplastic anemia, acquired and inherited. Philadelphia, PA: WB Saunders Co; 1993. p. 227-64.

[30] Patton W, Duffull S. Idiosyncratic drug-induced haematological abnormalities: incidence, pathogenosis, management, and avoidance. *Drug Safety,* 1994;11:445-462.

[31] Fausel C. Neutropenia and Agranulocytosis. Bethesda, MD: American Society of Health-System Pharmacists; 2005. P. 671-681.

[32] Shapiro S, Issaragrisil S, Kaufman DW, et al. Agranulocytosis in Bangkok, Thailand: a predominantly drug-induced disease with an unusually low incidence. Aplastic Anemia Study Group. *Am. J. trop. Med. Hyg.,* 1999;60:573-577.

[33] Van der Klauw M, Wilson J, Stricker B. Drug-associated agranulocytosis: 20 years of reporting in the Netherlands (1974-1994). *Am. J. Hematol.,* 1998;57:206-211.

[34] International Agranulocytosis and Aplastic Anaemia Study. Risk of agranulocytosis and aplastic anaemia in relation to use of antithyroid drugs. *BMJ,* 1988;297:262-265.

[35] Kelly JP, Kaufman DW, and Shapiro S. Risks of agranulocytosis and aplastic anemia in relation to the use of cardiovascular drugs: the International Agranulocytosis and Aplastic Anemia study. *Clin. Pharmacol. Ther.,* 1991;49:330-341.
[36] Anti-infective drug use in relation to the risk of agranulocytosis and aplastic anemia. A report from the International Agranulocytosis and Aplastic Anemia study. *Arch. Intern. Med.,* 1989;149:1036-1040.
[37] Rawson NS, Harding SR, Malcolm E, et al. Hospitalizations for aplastic anemia and agranulocytosis in Saskatchewan: incidence and associations with antecedent prescription drug use. *J. Clin. epidemiol.,* 1998;51:1343-1355.
[38] Van Staa TP, Boulton F, Cooper C, et al. Neutropenia and agranulocytosis in England and Wales: incidence and risk factors. *Am. J. Hematol.,* 2003;72:248-254.
[39] Claas FH. Immune mechanisms leading to drug-induced blood dyscrasias. *Eur. J. Haematol.,* 1996;60(supp):64-68.
[40] Levitt LJ. Chlorpropramid-induced pure white blood cell aplasia. *Blood,* 1987;69:394-400.
[41] Heit WF. Hematologic effects of antipyretic analgesics: drug-induced agranulocytosis. *Am. J. Med.,* 1983;75:65-68.
[42] Toth E, Mant M, Shivji S, et al. Propylthiouracil-induced agranulocytosis: an unusual presentation and a possible mechanism. *Am. J. Med.,* 1988;85:725-727.
[43] Wall J, Fang S, Kuroki T, et al. In vitro immunoreactivity to propylthiouracil, methimazole, and carbimazole in patients with Graves' disease: a possible cause of antithyroid drug-induced agranulocytosis. *J. Clin. Endocrinol. Metab.,* 1984;58:868-872.
[44] Guffy M, Goeken N, Burns C. Granulocytotoxic antibodies in a patient with prophylthiouracil-induced agranulocytosis. *Arch. Intern. Med.,* 1984;144:1687-1688.
[45] Fibbe W, Claas F, Van der Star-Dijkstra W, et al. Agranulocytosis induced by prophylthiouracil: evidence of a drug dependent antibody reacting with granulocytes, monocytes, and haematopoietic progenitor cells. *Br. J. Haematol.,* 1986;64:363-373.
[46] Guest I, Uetrecht J. Drugs that induce neutropenia/agranulocytosis may target specific componenet of the stromal cell extracellular matrix. *Med. Hypotheses,* 1999;53:145-151.
[47] Iverson S, Zahid N, Uetrecht J. Predicting drug-induced agranulocytosis: characterizing neutrophil-generated metabolites of a model compound,

DMP 406, and assessing the relevance of an in vitro apoptosis assay for identifying drugs that may cause agranulocytosis. *Chem. Biol. Interact.*, 2002;142:175-199.

[48] Ascensao J, Flynn P, Slungaard A, et al. Quinidine-induced neutropenia:report of a case with drug-dependent inhibition of granulocyte colony generation. *Acta Haemat.*, 1984;72:349-354.

[49] Fitchen J, Koeffler H. Cimetidine and granulopoiesis: bone marrow culture studies in normal man and patients with cimetidine-associated neutropenia. *Br. J. Haematol.*, 1980;46:361-366.

[50] Uetrecht J. Metabolism of clozapine by neutrophils. Possible implications for clozapine-induced agranulocytosis. *Drug Safety*, 1992;21:830-834.

[51] Williams D, Pirmohamed M, Naisbitt D, et al. Induction of metabolism dependent and independent neutrophil apoptosis by clozapine. *Mol. Pharmacol.*, 2000;58:207-216.

[52] Paitel J, Stockemer V, Dorvaux V, et al. Agranulocytoses aiguës médicamenteuses. Etude clinique à propos de 30 patients et évolution des étiologies sur 2 décennies. *Rev. Med. Interne*, 1995;16:495–9.

[53] Andrès E, Noel E, Kurtz J, et al. Life-threatening idiosyncratic drug-induced agranulocytosis in elderly patients. *Drugs Aging*, 2004;21:427–35.

[54] Kurtz JE, Andrès E, Maloisel F, et al. Drug-induced agranulocytosis in elderly. A case series of 25 patients. *Age Aging*, 1999;28:325–6.

[55] Tajiri J. Antithyroid drug-induced agranulocytosis: special reference to normal white cell count agranulocytosis. *Thyroid* 2004;14:459–62.

[56] Tajiri J, Noguchi S, Murakami T, et al. Antithyroid drug-induced agranulocytosis. The usefulness of routine white blood cell count monitoring. *Arch. Intern. Med.*, 1990;150:621–4.

[57] Shastri K, Logue G. Autoimmune neutropenia. *Blood*, 1993;81:1984–95.

[58] Dale D, Guerry I, Wewerka J, et al. Chronic neutropenia. *Medicine*, (Baltimore) 1979;58:128–44.

[59] Akhtari M, Curtis B, Waller E. Autoimmune neutropenia in adults. *Autoimmunity Reviews*, 2009;9:62-66.

[60] Akamizu T, Oaxaki S, Hiratani H, et al. Drug-induced neutropenia associated with anti-neutrophil cytoplasmic antibodies (ANCA): possible involvement of complement in granulocyte cyctotoxicity. *Clin. Exp. Immunol.*, 2002:127:92-98.

[61] Risks of agranulocytosis and aplastic anemia. A first report of their relation to drug use with special reference to analgesics. The

International Agranulocytosis and Aplastic Anemia Study. *JAMA,* 1986;256:1749-1757.

[62] Hedenmalm K, Spigset O. Agranulocytosis and other blood dyscrasias associated with dipyrone (metamizole). *Eur. J. Clin. Pharmcol.,* 2002; 58: 265-274.

[63] Keisu M, Ekman E. Sulfasalazine associated agranulocytosis in Sweden 1972-1989. Clinical features and estimation of its incidence. *Eur. J. Clin. Pharmacol.,* 1992;43:215-218.

[64] Andres E, Maloisel F, Zimmer J. The role of haematopoietic growth factors granulocyte colony-stimulating factor and granulocyte-macrophage colony-stimulating factor in the management of drug-induced agranulocytosis. *Br. J. Haematol.,* 2010;150:3-8.

[65] Andres E, Kurtz J, Perrin A, et al. The use of haematopoietic growth factors in antithyroid-related drug-induced agranulocytosis: a report of 20 patients. *Q. J. Med.*, 2001;94:423-428.

[66] Andres E, Kurtz J, Martin-Hunyadi C, et al. Non-chemotherapy drug-induced agranulocytosis in elderly patients: the effects of granulocyte colony-stimulating factor. *Am. J. Med.*, 2002;112:460-464.

[67] Freifeld A, Bow E, Sepkowitz K, et al. Clinical practice guideline for the use of antimicrobial agents in neutropenic patients with cancer: 2010 update by the Infectious Diseases Society of America. *CID*. 2011; 52:e56-e93.

[68] Maloisel F, Andres E, Kaltenbach G, et al. Prognostic factors of hematologic recovery in nonchemotherapy drug-induced agranulocytosis. *Haematologica*, 2003;88:470-471.

[69] Ibanez L, Sabate M, Ballarin E, et al. Use of granulocyte colony-stimulating factor (G-CSF) and outcome in patients with non-chemotherapy agranulocytosis. *Pharmacoepidemiol Drug Safety,* 2008;17:224-228.

[70] Fukata S, Kuma K, Sugawara M. Granulocyte colony-stimulating factor (G-CSF) does not improve recovery from anti-thyroid drug-induced agranulocytosis: a prospective study. *Thyroid,* 1999;9(1):29-31.

[71] Sprikkelman A, M. de Wolf J, Vellenga E. The application of hematopoietic growth factors in drug-induced agranulocytosis: a review of 70 cases. *Leukemia*, 1994; 8(12):2031-2036.

[72] Beauchesne M, Shalansky S. Nonchemotherapy drug-induced agranulocytosis: a review of 118 patients treated with colony-stimulating factors. *Pharmacotherapy*, 1999;19(3):299-305.

In: Neutropenia
Editors: M. Akhtari et al.
ISBN: 978-1-63482-105-6

Chapter 3

Neutropenia in Felty's Syndrome

Bryant England[1], Mohammad Bager Owlia[2] and Mojtaba Akhtari[3*]
[1]Division of Rheumatology, Department of Internal Medicine, Nebraska Medical Center, University of Nebraska Medical Center, Omaha, NE, US
[2]Department of Internal Medicine, Shahid Sadoughi University of Medical Sciences, Yazd, Iran
[3]Jane Anne Nohl Division of Hematology and Center for the Study of Blood Diseases, University of Southern California (USC)/ Norris Cancer Center, USC University Hospital, Keck Medical Center of USC, Los Angeles, CA, US

Introduction

Felty's syndrome (FS) is characterized by rheumatoid arthritis (RA) with accompanying neutropenia in the absence of other specific causes for the neutropenia. Splenomegaly, which was included in the original description of FS, is frequently observed but not required for diagnosis. Between 1 to 3% of individuals with RA have been reported to develop FS, but its prevalence among different centers and observations may differ. Classically, FS appears in individuals with severe RA usually after 10 years in duration. Extra-

* Corresponding author: Makhtari@usc.edu

articular manifestations are common in those who develop FS and joint destruction is usually quite severe despite the absence of active synovitis. Nearly all individuals with FS are positive for HLA-DR4 alleles and levels of rheumatoid factor, antinuclear antibodies, immune complexes, and immunoglobulins are elevated in the serum. As a result of the neutropenia, individuals with FS have increased risk of recurrent bacterial skin and respiratory tract infections. These infections are usually seen when the absolute neutrophil count (ANC) falls below 100 cells/μL. The pathogenesis leading to neutropenia in FS is complex and multifactorial, with cellular and humoral immune responses contributing. Immune mediated destruction of circulating neutrophils is the driving factor, but there is evidence of neutrophil activation and sequestration as well as bone marrow changes such as maturation arrest of myeloid progenitor cells that contribute to neutropenia. Treatment is not mandatory for asymptomatic individuals with FS whose neutropenia is not severe, but is indicated when ANC falls to below 500 cells/μL or when an infection occurs. The first-line treatment for FS is use of disease modifying anti-rheumatic drugs (DMARDs). Methotrexate (MTX) and intramuscular gold have the most support for their use in the literature though MTX has largely replaced the use of gold in FS. For neutropenia not responding to DMARDs, granulocyte colony-stimulating factor has been shown to improve neutrophil counts. Splenectomy may be indicated in cases refractory to pharmacologic therapy. Normalization of neutrophil count is seen in nearly all individuals within 48 hours following splenectomy, though 25% have recurrent neutropenia. Approximately 40% of individuals with FS develop large granular lymphocyte (LGL) syndrome, which consists of a polyclonal proliferation of CD3+, CD8+, CD57+ T-cells. Systemic prednisone along with MTX is the first-line therapy for LGL, with cyclosporine A, cyclophosphamide, colony stimulating factors and biological agents as other available options. Splenectomy may be indicated in cases refractory to other therapies and is of less benefit in LGL than in FS.

Background

Felty's Syndrome (FS) was first reported by AR Felty in 1924 at John's Hopkins Hospital in five patients with the triad of rheumatoid arthritis (RA), neutropenia, and splenomegaly [1]. FS is an extra-articular manifestation of RA and typically develops approximately 10 to 15 years after the onset of RA

[2]. Between 1 to 3% of those with RA are reported to develop FS [2, 3]. However, none of 613 cases of RA in a series from two clinic sites in Iran were complicated with FS [4]. Furthermore, some experts argue that improved treatment of RA has likely reduced the progression to FS. While originally splenomegaly was felt to be an essential component of FS, clinical similarity between those with and without splenomegaly lead to its elimination as an essential component of the diagnostic criteria [5]. The criterion for diagnosis of FS is generally felt to consist of RA with persistent neutropenia not attributable to other causes. There is no set degree of neutropenia required for diagnosis and review of the literature displays different values in each study. The severity of neutropenia in FS fluctuates and in some instances spontaneously remits [5].

Disease Characteristics

Clinical

The arthritis in FS is generally quite severe. Erosive changes are seen on radiographs and in some instances there is an absence of active synovitis [5, 6]. Extra-articular findings are common including anemia, rheumatoid nodules, leg ulcers, hepatomegaly, and hepatic histiologic abnormalities such as nodular regenerative hyperplasia [7, 8]. There are some reports of FS without RA, indicating a possible distinct entity for FS [9].

Serum

While RA has a strong association with HLA-DR4, FS has an even stronger association, being found in greater than 90% of those with FS [5, 10]. This increased frequency of DR4 is primarily due to the presence of subtype Dw4 (0401) [11]. Almost all serologic markers in FS are more striking than the classic RA and this serologic resemblance of FS to systemic lupus erythemetosus (SLE) possibly makes FS a condition closer to SLE spectrum rather than RA. Rheumatoid factor (RF) is also found in higher prevalence in FS than RA with studies reporting between 90 to 100% of those with FS seropositive for RF [8, 12]. Anti-cyclic citrulinated peptide antibodies (ACPA) were reported in 74% of FS in a recent study composed of sera from 23 patients [13]. Due to scarcity of new evidence, further data on ACPA in FS is lacking. Antinuclear antibody (ANA) positivity is seen in approximately 60% of FS and anti-histone antibodies in about 70%. Antibodies to SSA, SSB, U1RNP, Smith are not usually found in the sera of patients with FS [5].

Infections

Approximately 60% of individuals with FS will have an infection attributable to neutropenia. The skin and respiratory tract are common sites for infection and often these infections are recurrent. Goldberg combined data from 90 patients with FS and found the sites of infections to be skin (26%), respiratory (24%), urinary tract (9%), buccal ulcers (4%), sinusitis/otitis (4%), and septic arthritis (2%) [2]. Causative bacterial organisms are Staphylococcus, Streptococcus, Haemophilus, and gram negative bacilli [8]. In a prospective long-term outcome study by Thorne, five-year mortality in FS was 36% with infections being the leading cause-of-death [14]. Similarly, Campion followed FS patients for five years and found a mortality of 25% with sepsis being the leading cause-of-death. Though neutropenia places individuals with FS at increased risk of infection, the degree of neutropenia does not correlate well with the risk of infection until counts are markedly low (absolute neutrophil count [ANC] <100) [5]. Low Fc receptor III and high G-CSF levels correlate with the rate of infection better than ANC [15]. Due to the established role of infections in inducing neutropenia, a major dilemma would be differentiation of primary versus secondary infections in similar clinical settings.

Pathogenesis

The pathophysiology behind FS is complex and multifactorial. While multiple theories have been proposed, the exact mechanisms remain unknown. Established mechanisms for developing neutropenia include: (1) excessive margination, (2) increased sequestration or peripheral destruction, and (3) impaired granulopoiesis [16]. The evidence for each of these mechanisms in FS is presented individually.

Excessive Margination

Data is conflicting regarding the contribution of excessive margination of neutrophils to neutropenia in FS. Vincent et al. studied neutrophil kinetics in seventeen FS patients. All showed evidence of excessive margination of neutrophils; in 12 of the 17 patients, excessive margination explained the complete decrease in neutrophil count. In two patients who underwent splenectomy, margination of neutrophils was decreased following the procedure [17]. Joyce et al. also studied neutrophil kinetics in 19 FS patients and while they observed accelerated marrow release and disappearance of mature neutrophils, they found no evidence for increased margination [18].

Increased Sequestration and Peripheral Destruction

Increased sequestration and peripheral destruction of neutrophils appears to be the driving force behind neutropenia in FS. This occurs secondary to the interaction between neutrophils and circulating immune complexes. While immunoglobulins bind to the surface of neutrophils in FS, this interaction is not mediated by the Fab fragment [19, 20]. Rather, immune complexes are adherent to the Fc fragment, C3b, or are phagocytosed by neutrophils resulting in surface changes leading to increased sequestration and destruction [19, 21]. A possible antigenic target of these antibodies is Eukaryotic elongation factor 1A-1 (Anti-eeF1A1). Anti-eeF1A1 was found in sera of 66% FS patients in one study and strongly correlated with ANA [22].

A newly proposed mechanism of neutrophil cell death in FS is production of neutrophil extracellular chromatin traps or NETosis. Autoantibodies against PAD-4-deiminated histones in activated neutrophils and NETs have been demonstrated in FS. It is proposed the production of these autoantibodies further activates neutrophils leading to depletion of mature neutrophils [13].

Impaired Granulopoiesis

In addition to peripheral destruction, there appears to be impaired granulopoiesis contributing to the neutropenia in FS. Autoantibodies to Granulocyte-colony stimulating factors (G-CSF) have been found in the serum of FS patients. In many of the individuals these antibodies had neutralizing capabilities. Furthermore, bone marrow in FS patients has decreased responsiveness to G-CSF [23]. Decreased in vitro growth of immature granulocytes (Colony-Forming Unit Culture) has been observed in FS [2]. Colony stimulating activity (CSA) has been measured in the urine and serum of FS patients and levels were found to be decreased in both, relative to controls [2, 24]. Bucknall et al. showed decreased marrow neutrophil reserves in RA with neutropenia [6]. Both cell-mediated and non-immunoglobulin humoral factors suppress normal granulopoiesis [25].

Bone marrow characteristics of patients with FS have been described in many studies. The majority of studies show maturation arrest of myeloid progenitor cells. The cellularity of the bone marrow typically is normocellular or hypercellular, though hypocellular marrow has been reported [2, 5, 8]. Example bone marrow slides from patients with FS are shown in Figure 1.

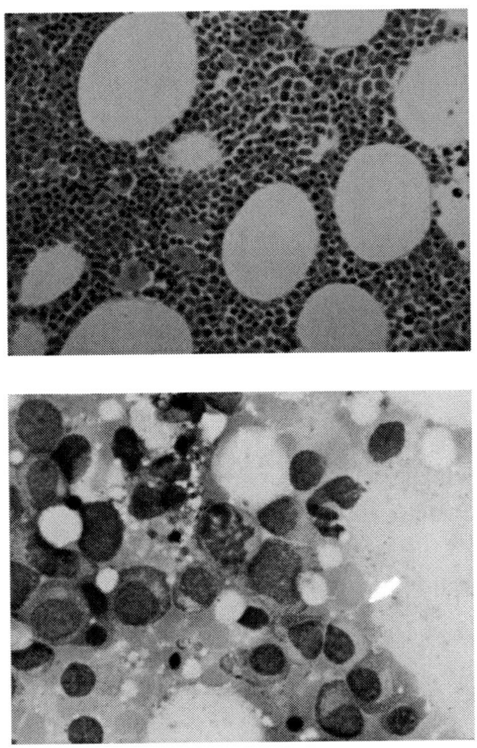

Figure 1. Bone marrow slides of Felty's syndrome patients.
Top figure: Hypercellular bone marrow biopsy from a patient with Felty's syndrome.
Bottom figure: Large granular lymphocyte in bone marrow aspiration from a patient with Felty's syndrome (Arrow).

An illustration of the mechanisms of neutropenia in FS is shown in Figure 2.

Treatment

There are no randomized controlled trials evaluating therapies for neutropenia in FS. The literature consists of case reports and a small number of retrospective studies. Furthermore, there is no standard for determining a successful treatment response. Goals when treating neutropenia should be increasing neutrophil count, preventing infectious complications, and limiting potential side effects. Disease modifying anti-rheumatic drugs (DMARDs) such as methotrexate, gold, cyclosporine, cyclophosphamide, D-penicillamine, hydroxychloroquine, and leflunomide all have evidence to support their use. Other treatments that have been reported include lithium carbonate, colony stimulating factors, and splenectomy. Case reports do not support the use of etanercept in treating neutropenia in FS. Evidence for each therapy is described individually.

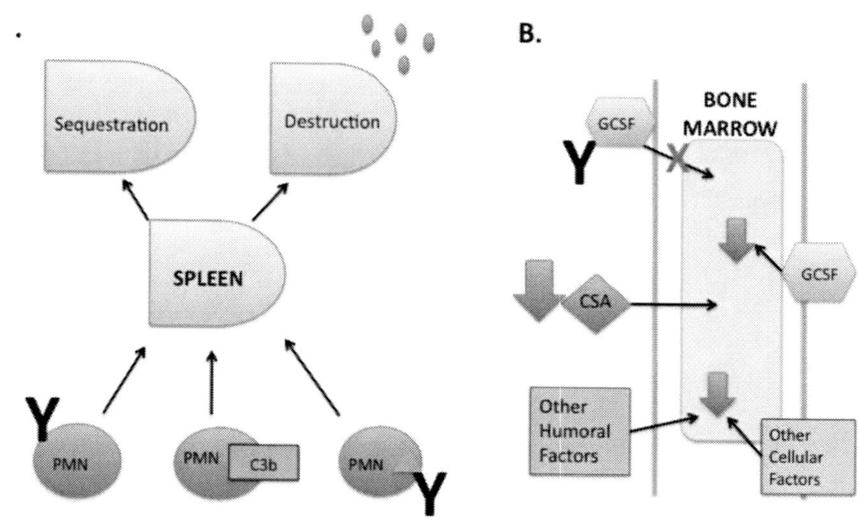

Figure 2. Mechansim of neutropenia in Felty's syndrome. (A) Binding of PMN to Fc receptor, binding of PMN to C3b, phagocytosis of immune complex by PMN leading to surface changes resulting in splenic sequestration and destruction. (B) Antibody binding to G-CSF, decreased bone marrow responsiveness to G-CSF, decreased CSA, suppression of bone marrow function by other humoral and cellular factors.

Corticosteroids

Low dose corticosteroids have not been shown to raise neutrophil counts in FS. Higher doses may increase neutrophil count, but this improvement does not persist if dose is decreased or therapy is discontinued [12]. Corticosteroids do not decrease the rate of infection and in fact, long-term use with higher doses was found to be associated with an increased rate of infection [26]. Many of the case reports reviewed used corticosteroids as adjuvant therapy and it appears this is the main role for corticosteroids in FS, in addition to controlling joint symptoms such as synovitis.

Methotrexate

Methotrexate (MTX) is generally considered to be the first-line therapy for the treatment of neutropenia in FS. There are no randomized controlled trials evaluating its efficacy; the data consists of case reports as well as a retrospective study by Wassenberg et al. Upon retrospective analysis, neutrophil count was significantly elevated in seven patients treated with methotrexate after one year. The average dose of methotrexate used was 12.86 mg and no side effects limiting its use occurred. Furthermore, joint symptoms and ESR decreased over the follow-up period. Wassenberg et al. also reviewed the previous case reports in the literature where methotrexate was used. Twelve of thirteen cases had improvement in neutrophil count with follow-up ranging from three weeks to twelve years [27]. While the data is limited and biased, the excellent response seen, the fact MTX is well tolerated, and the success of MTX in RA have lead to its widespread use in FS.

Colony Stimulating Factors

Colony stimulating factors are effective at raising neutrophil counts. Side effects limit their use and resolution of neutropenia is dependent on continuing with therapy. Thus, their use is best in situations where a short-term elevation of neutrophil count is needed. Stanworth et al. prospectively studied eight patients, most who had recurrent infections, who were treated with G-CSF. Six of the patients had side effects that caused them to discontinue use, decrease the dose, or switch formulations. Joint pains were a common complaint, but long-term use of G-CSF did not affect disease activity score. Neutrophil counts improved and rates of infections decreased in the five patients who were maintained on G-CSF [28]. Hellmich et al. also studied a group of FS patients treated with G-CSF. Three of the five patients had improvement in neutrophil count. Furthermore, they reviewed 42 prior cases of treatment with G-CSF; all cases reported significant improvements in neutrophil count. The most common side effect reported was bone pain, which was seen in 20% of patients [29]. Hazenberg reported a case of FS treated with GM-CSF with improvement in neutrophil count over 14 days of therapy; however, the patient did have worsening of joint pain and increased serum levels of cytokines [30].

Splenectomy

Historically, the first-line treatment for neutropenia in FS was splenectomy, which was first performed in 1932 [31]. Short-term results are excellent as the neutrophil count rises rapidly and consistently following surgery [32, 33]. A review of retrospective studies by Rashba revealed a response rate of 80% following splenectomy [34]. Long-term results are not as robust. In a prospective study with an average five-year follow-up, 50% of patients who underwent splenectomy had recurrent infections [14]. While there is a rise in neutrophil count after splenectomy, the lack of evidence for prevention of future infections as well as the complications associated with splenectomy has resulted in it being considered a therapy of last resort.

Hydroxychloroquine

Two patients successfully treated with hydroxychloroquine (HCQ) were reported by Mahevas et al. The first developed hepatitis and thrombocytopenia after initiation of MTX. After starting HCQ, neutrophil count and arthritis improved throughout 22 months of follow-up until the patient discontinued the medication. Subsequently, both the arthritis flared and neutrophil count sharply declined. Upon re-institution of hydroxychloroquine, neutrophil count and arthritis improved. The second patient remained neutropenic despite the use of methotrexate for one year. Peripheral blood samples revealed T-cell large granular lymphocyte (TLGL) proliferation. Neutrophil count normalized within four months after starting HCQ and remained within normal ranges for two years [35].

Cyclosporine

Canvin reported a case of FS treated with cyclosporine after failing therapy with cyclophosphamide. Neutrophil count improved by six weeks and normalized after three months of therapy. Tapering the dose resulted in decline in neutrophil count and an infection. Neutrophil count responded once the dose was increased again [36]. Coiffier reported a case of FS with profound neutropenia, ANC 0, and infectious complications which did not respond to treatment with lithium but responded well to treatment with cyclosporine. Neutrophil count began to rise within four weeks and normalized by two months. Throughout eight months of follow-up, neutrophil counts remained elevated. Infectious complications persisted for the first month of therapy then resolved throughout the duration of follow-up [37].

Cyclophosphamide

There are two case reports demonstrating efficacy of cyclophosphamide increasing neutrophil counts, one independently and one prior to administering G-CSF. Neish and Fuchs reported a case of FS with neutropenia successfully treated with cyclophosphamide as monotherapy [38]. Pixley et al. reported a case of FS complicated by recurrent infections and sepsis where cyclophosphamide was used prior to administering G-CSF. This treatment combination successfully treated the neutropenia and actually produced a neutrophilia [39].

Rituximab

Results are mixed regarding the efficacy of rituximab, a monoclonal antibody to CD20, in treating neutropenia in FS. Weinreb et al. reported a case of FS refractory to treatment with multiple DMARDs, infliximab, prednisone, and G-CSF. Following administration of rituximab, HCQ and prednisone, neutrophil count, inflammatory markers and reported pain improved throughout nine months of follow-up [40]. Lekharaju and Chattopadhyay reported a similar case of refractory FS. Disease activity score, erythrocyte sedimentation rate (ESR), and neutrophil count improved following administration of a single dose of rituximab in combination with MTX and prednisone; this benefit persisted throughout 14 months of follow-up [41]. In contrast, Sordet et al. reported two cases of FS refractory to DMARDs where neutrophil count, disease activity, and inflammatory markers did not respond to four doses of weekly rituximab over a six-month follow-up. One patient was receiving concurrent MTX therapy and both were receiving corticosteroids [42]. Salama et al. reported a case of refractory FS where the arthritis and hemolysis improved after initiation of rituximab, but no improvement in neutrophil count was observed [43]. With conflicting case reports in the literature, one can only conclude rituximab may be beneficial in the treatment of neutropenia in refractory FS.

D-penicillamine

Lakhanpal reported data from eight patients with FS treated with D-penicillamine for a mean of one year. Cutaneous ulcers healed in four of six patients. Recurrent infections resolved in three of five patients. However, D-penicillamine was discontinued in six patients due to lack of efficacy or side effects. One patient developed pancytopenia and died [44].

Leflunomide

There is one case report suggesting leflunomide is beneficial in FS. Talip et al. reported a case of FS with neutropenia refractory to treatment with HCQ, parenteral gold, MTX, prednisone, and etanercept. G-CSF produced a transient increase in neutrophil count. After starting therapy with leflunomide, neutrophil count gradually improved over six months. Arthritic symptoms improved and leg ulcerations healed [45].

Etanercept

There is no evidence that etanercept, a tumor necrosis factor-α (TNF-α) inhibitor, is effective in treating neutropenia in FS. Ghavami reported a case of FS refractory to azathioprine and corticosteroids treated with etanercept. Therapy was initiated because of increasing synovitis. While joint symptoms and inflammatory markers improved, neutrophil count declined markedly over 14 months and the patient experienced an episode of septic arthritis. Etanercept was discontinued and MTX was started resulting in normalization of neutrophil count within three months [46]. Ravindran also reported a case of FS in a patient with Sjogrens syndrome and amyloidosis. Neutrophil count did not improve following treatment with etanercept [47].

Historic Drugs

Both lithium carbonate and gold salts have been used historically to treat FS [48-51]. Both medications have now been replaced by newer DMARD agents. It is proposed lithium carbonate stimulated production of CSA [52]. The mechanism of action of gold salts is unknown.

The different treatments as well as the evidence to support their use are summarized in Table 1.

Table 1. Summary of treatment options for neutropenia in FS

Treatment	Mechanism of Action	Advantages	Disadvantages
Methotrexate	Inhibits folate metabolism inducing apoptosis in activated lymphocytes	Several case reports with successful treatment of neutropenia Has been used extensively and effectively in RA	No prospective studies have been performed
Corticoste-roids	Bind to glucocorticoid receptor which then attach to DNA promoter sequence leading to transcription of anti-inflammatory proteins	High doses can increase neutrophil count Used as adjunctive therapy in many studies	Low dose steroids do not increase neutrophil count Higher dose of steroids correlates with higher rates of infections
Colony Stimulating Factors	Stimulate proliferation and maturation of immature neutrophils	Effective at raising neutrophil counts in several studies Infection rate decreased in one study Raise neutrophil count within a couple weeks	Side effects limit use May cause joint symptoms to worsen

Treatment	Mechanism of Action	Advantages	Disadvantages
Splenectomy	Prevents sequestration of neutrophils and removal of neutrophils by spleen	Rapid and near universal rise in neutrophils following procedure	Not proven to decrease rate of infection Complications with procedure
Hydroxychlo-roquine	Reduces activation of antigen presenter cells, suppresses leukocyte response, inhibition of neutrophil chemotaxis, among others	Neutropenia improved in two case reports	Neutrophil counts fell once therapy discontinued
Cyclosporine	Prevents activation and proliferation of T-cells	Neutropenia improved in two case reports Infections resolved in one patient	Neutrophil counts fell in one patient when dose decreased
Cyclophos-phamide	Alkylating agent suppressing T-cell activation and inducing T-cell apoptosis	Neutropenia improved in two case reports	Was used in combination with G-CSF in one case to achieve response
Rituximab	Monoclonal antibody to CD20 on B-cells	Neutrophil counts improved in two studies when rituximab was used in combination with HCQ or MTX	Two case reports showed no improvement to neutrophil count with rituximab No evidence sole therapy with rituximab increases neutrophil count
D-penicilla-mine	Unknown	Infections decreased in about 50% of subjects	Side effects and lack of efficacy lead to discontinuation in most subjects One patient developed pancytopenia and died
Leflunomide	Pyrimidine synthesis inhibitor preventing expansion of activated lymphocytes	Neutropenia and infections improved in one case	Only one case report in literature

Large Granular Lymphocytes

Characteristics

Approximately 40% of individuals with FS have evidence of large granular lymphocytes in the serum [53]. TLGL leukemia is a clonal proliferation of cytotoxic T-lymphocytes (CTL) expressing a typical immunophenotype of CD3+, CD8+, CD57+. Major clinical characteristics consist of neutropenia, frequent infections, anemia, and RA. About 25% of individuals with TLGL have RA, with RA usually preceding the diagnosis of TLGL [54]. FS and TLGL share characteristics such as RA and neutropenia, which makes them difficult to distinguish. Currently, these disorders are distinguished by the presence of T-cell clonality. This is determined by PCR amplification of the TCR-γ gene, which is present in TLGL but not in FS [55]. Clinical differences between the two disorders include synovitis, joint destruction, and circulating RF which are much more prevalent in FS [16]. Extra-articular manifestations such as leg ulcers, hepatomegaly, and splenomegaly also are seen much more frequently in FS than TLGL [55].

As mentioned above the similarity of clinical features suggests a link between the two diseases. Furthermore, genetic analysis provides more insight into the spectrum of these diseases. Bowman et al. have shown the frequency of shared epitope positive HLA-DR4 allelles in individuals with TLGL and RA is similar to individuals with FS, at about 80-90% [56]. Coakley et al. found FS and TLGL with RA to have identical MHC class II associations, as well as a strong primary association with HLA-DRB1*0401 [57].

Pathogenesis

There is strong evidence that neutropenia associated with TLGL is mediated by Fas-ligand. Fas-ligand is elevated in the sera of patients with TLGL and TLGL cells are resistant to Fas-mediated apoptosis [58, 59]. Burks and Loughran proposed that excess Fas-ligand results in an induction of apoptosis of immature myeloid elements with reduced proliferation and differentiation. Ultimately, the result is a bone marrow proliferation defect resulting from the accumulation of CTL [55].

Treatment

MTX is considered the first-line therapy for TLGL. An uncontrolled, prospective study of 10 patients showed a complete response, defined as normal blood counts and CD3+ lymphocytes, in five patients. Time to achieve an ANC > 500 was between two weeks and four months. [60]. Cyclosporin A is also effective at reversing the neutropenia associated with TLGL, though it does not normalize lymphocytes [61]. Dhodapkar reported similar rates of successful treatment of neutropenia with prednisone as sole therapy and cyclophosphamide with adjunctive prednisone [62]. Corticosteroids, however, are most commonly used as adjunctive therapy. Colony stimulating factors have been shown to increase neutrophil count in TLGL, but upon cessation of therapy, all counts fell to pre-treatment values [63]. Splenectomy improved neutrophil counts in all four patients studied, but only two achieved sustained response, all had increased levels of LGL, and one died of an accelerated lymphoproliferative disorder 19 months following splenectomy [64].

Key Points

- Felty's syndrome (FS) is seen in a subset of patients with longstanding rheumatoid arthritis (RA) and is defined by RA and neutropenia.
- Because of neutropenia, individuals with FS have increased rates of infections
- Pathogenesis is complex, but is driven by immune complex mediated destruction and sequestration of neutrophils.
- Methotrexate is the first-line therapy for FS; other effective treatments include other DMARDs, colony stimulating factors, corticosteroids, and splenectomy.
- A subset of FS may have clonal proliferation of cytotoxic T-cells known as T-cell large granular lymphocytes (TLGL).
- TLGL and FS lie on the same spectrum of disease.

References

[1] Felty AR. Chronic arthritis in the adult, associated with splenomegaly and leucopenia: A report of five cases of an unusual clinical syndrome. *Bulletin of Johns Hopkins Hospital*. 1924;35:16-20.

[2] Goldberg J, Pinals RS. Felty syndrome. *Semin Arthritis Rheum*. 1980;10(1):52-65.

[3] Sibley JT, Haga M, Visram DA, Mitchell DM. The clinical course of felty's syndrome compared to matched controls. *J Rheumatol*. 1991;18(8):1163-1167.

[4] Bagher OM, Golbarg M, Hossein S. Pattern of rheumatic diseases in two outpatient clinics in iran: Similarities with some different features. *Indian J Med Sci*. 2011;65(1):7-17. doi: 10.4103/0019-5359.103160; 10.4103/0019-5359.103160.

[5] Campion G, Maddison PJ, Goulding N, et al. The felty syndrome: A case-matched study of clinical manifestations and outcome, serologic features, and immunogenetic associations. *Medicine (Baltimore)*. 1990;69(2):69-80.

[6] Bucknall RC, Davis P, Bacon PA, Jones JV. Neutropenia in rheumatoid arthritis: Studies on possible contributing factors. *Ann Rheum Dis*. 1982;41(3):242-247.

[7] Thorne C, Urowitz MB, Wanless I, Roberts E, Blendis LM. Liver disease in felty's syndrome. *Am J Med*. 1982;73(1):35-40.

[8] Sienknecht CW, Urowitz MB, Pruzanski W, Stein HB. Felty's syndrome. clinical and serological analysis of 34 cases. *Ann Rheum Dis*. 1977;36(6):500-507.

[9] Rozin A, Hoffman R, Hayek T, Balbir-Gurman A. Felty's syndrome without rheumatoid arthritis?. *Clin Rheumatol*. 2013. doi: 10.1007/s10067-012-2157-3.

[10] Friman C, Schlaut J, Davis P. HLA-DR4 in felty's syndrome. *J Rheumatol*. 1985;12(3):628-629.

[11] Lanchbury JSS, Jaeger EEM, Sansom DM, et al. Strong primary selection for the Dw4 subtype of DR4 accounts for the HLA-DQw7 association with felty's syndrome. *Hum Immunol*. 1991;32(1):56-64. doi: 10.1016/0198-8859(91)90117-R.

[12] Barnes CG, Turnbull AL, Vernon-Roberts B. Felty's syndrome. A clinical and pathological survey of 21 patients and their response to treatment. *Ann Rheum Dis*. 1971;30(4):359-374.

[13] Dwivedi N, Upadhyay J, Neeli I, et al. Felty's syndrome autoantibodies bind to deiminated histones and neutrophil extracellular chromatin traps. *Arthritis Rheum*. 2012;64(4):982-992. doi: 10.1002/art.33432; 10.1002/art.33432.

[14] Thorne C, Urowitz MB. Long-term outcome in felty's syndrome. *Ann Rheum Dis*. 1982;41(5):486-489.

[15] Hellmich B, Csernok E, de Haas M, et al. Low fcgamma receptor III and high granulocyte colony-stimulating factor serum levels correlate with the risk of infection in neutropenia due to felty's syndrome or systemic lupus erythematosus. *Am J Med*. 2002;113(2):134-139.

[16] Rosenstein ED, Kramer N. Felty's and pseudo-felty's syndromes. *Semin Arthritis Rheum*. 1991;21(3):129-142.

[17] Vincent PC, Levi JA, Macqueen A. The mechanism of neutropenia in felty's syndrome. *Br J Haematol*. 1974;27(3):463-475.

[18] Joyce RA, Boggs DR, Chervenick PA, Lalezari P. Neutrophil kinetics in felty's syndrome. *Am J Med*. 1980;69(5):695-702.

[19] Breedveld FC, Lafeber GJ, Doekes G, Claas FH, Cats A. Felty syndrome: Autoimmune neutropenia or immune-complex-mediated disease?. *Rheumatol Int*. 1985;5(6):253-258.

[20] Petersen J, Wiik A. Lack of evidence for granulocyte specific membrane-directed autoantibodies in neutropenic cases of rheumatoid arthritis and in autoimmune neutropenia. *Acta Pathol Microbiol Immunol Scand C*. 1983;91(1):15-22.

[21] Hurd ER, Andreis M, Ziff M. Phagocytosis of immune complexes by polymorphonuclear leucocytes in patients with felty's syndrome. *Clin Exp Immunol*. 1977;28(3):413-425.

[22] Ditzel HJ, Masaki Y, Nielsen H, Farnaes L, Burton DR. Cloning and expression of a novel human antibody - antigen pair associated with felty's syndrome. *Proc Natl Acad Sci U S A*. 2000;97(16):9234-9239.

[23] Hellmich B, Csernok E, Schatz H, Gross WL, Schnabel A. Autoantibodies against granulocyte colony-stimulating factor in felty's syndrome and neutropenic systemic lupus erythematosus. *Arthritis Rheum*. 2002;46(9):2384-2391. doi: 10.1002/art.10497.

[24] Gupta R, Robinson WA, Albrecht D. Granulopoietic activity in felty's syndrome. *Ann Rheum Dis*. 1975;34(2):156-161.

[25] Starkebaum G, Singer JW, Arend WP. Humoral and cellular immune mechanisms of neutropenia in patients with felty's syndrome. *Clin Exp Immunol*. 1980;39(2):307-314.

[26] Breedveld FC, Fibbe WE, Hermans J, van der Meer JWM, Cats A. Factors influencing the incidence of infections in felty's syndrome. *Arch Intern Med*. 1987;147(5):915.

[27] Wassenberg S, Herborn G, Rau R. Methotrexate treatment in felty's syndrome. *Br J Rheumatol*. 1998;37(8):908-911.

[28] Stanworth SJ, Bhavnani M, Chattopadhya C, Miller H, Swinson DR. Treatment of felty's syndrome with the haemopoietic growth factor granulocyte colony-stimulating factor (G-CSF). *QJM Mon J Assoc Phys*. 1998;91(1):49-56.

[29] Hellmich B, Schnabel A, Gross WL. Treatment of severe neutropenia due to felty's syndrome or systemic lupus erythematosus with granulocyte colony-stimulating factor. *Semin Arthritis Rheum*. 1999;29(2):82-99.

[30] Hazenberg BPC, Van Leeuwen MA, Van Rijswijk MH, Stern AC, Vellenga E. Correction of granulocytopenia in felty's syndrome by granulocyte-macrophage colony-stimulating factor. simultaneous induction of interleukin-6 release and flare-up of the arthritis. *Blood*. 1989;74(8):2769-2770.

[31] Hanrahan EM MS. Effect of splenectomy in felty's syndrome. *JAMA*. 1932;99:1247.

[32] Spencer RP. Possible feedback control of white blood cells: Effect of splenectomy in felty's syndrome. *Med Hypotheses*. 1998;50(5):415-418.

[33] Riley SM, Aldrete JS. Role of splenectomy in felty's syndrome. *Am J Surg*. 1975;130(1):51-52.

[34] Rashba EJ, Rowe JM, Packman CH. Treatment of the neutropenia of felty syndrome. *Blood Rev*. 1996;10(3):177-184.

[35] Mahevas M, Audia S, De Lastours V, Michel M, Bonotte B, Godeau B. Neutropenia in felty's syndrome successfully treated with hydroxychloroquine. *Haematologica*. 2007;92(7):e78-9.

[36] Canvin JMG, Dalal BI, Baragar F, Johnston JB. Cyclosporine for the treatment of granulocytopenia in felty's syndrome. *Am J Hematol*. 1991;36(3):219-220.

[37] Coiffier B. Cyclosporine in felty's syndrome. *N Engl J Med*. 1986;314(3):184.

[38] Neish P.R. FHA. Resolution of felty's syndrome with cyclophosphamide. *Journal of Rheumatology*. 1989;16(5):709-710.

[39] Pixley JS, Yoneda KY, Manalo PB. Sequential administration of cyclophosphamide and granulocyte-colony stimulating factor relieves

impaired myeloid maturation in felty's syndrome. *Am J Hematol.* 1993;43(4):304-306.
[40] Weinreb N, Rabinowitz A, Dellaripa PF. Beneficial response to rituximab in refractory felty syndrome 2]. *J Clin Rheumatol.* 2006;12(1):48.
[41] Lekharaju V, Chattopadhyay C. Efficacy of rituximab in felty's syndrome. *Ann Rheum Dis.* 2008;67(9):1352.
[42] Sordet C, Gottenberg JE, Hellmich B, Kieffer P, Mariette X, Sibilia J. Lack of efficacy of rituximab in felty's syndrome. *Ann Rheum Dis.* 2005;64(2):332-333. doi: 10.1136/ard.2004.025643.
[43] Salama A, Schneider U, Dorner T. Beneficial response to rituximab in a patient with haemolysis and refractory felty syndrome. *Ann Rheum Dis.* 2008;67(6):894-895.
[44] Lakhanpal S, Luthra HS. D-penicillamine in felty's syndrome. *J Rheumatol.* 1985;12(4):703-706.
[45] Talip F, Walker N, Khan W, Zimmermann B. Treatment of felty's syndrome with leflunomide. *J Rheumatol.* 2001;28(4):868-870.
[46] Ghavami A, Genevay S, Fulpius T, Gabay C. Etanercept in treatment of felly's syndrome. *Ann Rheum Dis.* 2005;64(7):1090-1091.
[47] Ravindran J, Shenker N, Bhalla AK, Lachmann H, Hawkins P. Case report: Response in proteinuria due to AA amyloidosis but not felty's syndrome in a patient with rheumatoid arthritis treated with TNF-alpha blockade. *Rheumatology (Oxford).* 2004;43(5):669-672. doi: 10.1093/rheumatology/keh128.
[48] Gupta RC, Robinson WA, Smyth CJ. Efficacy of lithium in rheumatoid arthritis with granulocytopenia (felty's syndrome). A preliminary report. *Arthritis Rheum.* 1975;18(2):179-184.
[49] Mant MJ, Akabutu JJ, Herbert FA. Lithium carbonate therapy in severe felty's syndrome. benefits, toxicity, and granulocyte function. *Arch Intern Med.* 1986;146(2):277-280.
[50] Dillon AM, Luthra HS, Conn DL, Ferguson RH. Parenteral gold therapy in the felty syndrome. experience with 20 patients. *Medicine (Baltimore).* 1986;65(2):107-112.
[51] Almoallim H, Klinkhoff A. Longterm outcome of treatment of felty's syndrome with intramuscular gold: Case reports and recommendations for management. *J Rheumatol.* 2005;32(1):20-26.
[52] Robinson WA, Entringer MA, Huber J, Gupta R. In vivo and in vitro effects of lithium on granulopoiesis in human neutropenic disorders. *Adv Exp Med Biol.* 1980;127:281-291.

[53] Bowman SJ, Bhavnani M, Geddes GC, et al. Large granular lymphocyte expansions in patients with felty's syndrome: Analysis using anti-T cell receptor V(beta)-specific monoclonal antibodies. *Clin Exp Immunol.* 1995;101(1):18-24.

[54] Lamy T, Loughran T.P. J. Large granular lymphocyte leukemia. *Cancer Control.* 1998;5(1):25-33.

[55] Burks EJ, Loughran TP, Jr. Pathogenesis of neutropenia in large granular lymphocyte leukemia and felty syndrome. *Blood Rev.* 2006;20(5):245-266. doi: 10.1016/j.blre.2006.01.003.

[56] Bowman SJ, Sivakumaran M, Snowden N, et al. The large granular lymphocyte syndrome with rheumatoid arthritis. immunogenetic evidence for a broader definition of felty's syndrome. *Arthritis Rheum.* 1994;37(9):1326-1330.

[57] Coakley G, Brooks D, Iqbal M, et al. Major histocompatility complex haplotypic associations in felty's syndrome and large granular lymphocyte syndrome are secondary to allelic association with HLA-DRB1 *0401. *Rheumatology (Oxford).* 2000;39(4):393-398.

[58] Perzova R, Loughran TP, Jr. Constitutive expression of fas ligand in large granular lymphocyte leukaemia. *Br J Haematol.* 1997;97(1):123-126.

[59] Liu JH, Wei S, Lamy T, et al. Chronic neutropenia mediated by fas ligand. *Blood.* 2000;95(10):3219-3222.

[60] Loughran TP, Jr, Kidd PG, Starkebaum G. Treatment of large granular lymphocyte leukemia with oral low-dose methotrexate. *Blood.* 1994;84(7):2164-2170.

[61] Sood R, Stewart CC, Aplan PD, et al. Neutropenia associated with T-cell large granular lymphocyte leukemia: Long-term response to cyclosporine therapy despite persistence of abnormal cells. *Blood.* 1998;91(9):3372-3378.

[62] Dhodapkar MV, Li CY, Lust JA, Tefferi A, Phyliky RL. Clinical spectrum of clonal proliferations of T-large granular lymphocytes: A T-cell clonopathy of undetermined significance?. *Blood.* 1994;84(5):1620-1627.

[63] Mulder AB, de Wolf JT, Smit JW, van Oostveen JW, Vellenga E. Correction of neutropenia by GM-CSF in patients with a large granular lymphocyte proliferation. *Ann Hematol.* 1992;65(2):91-95.

[64] Loughran TP, Jr, Starkebaum G, Clark E, Wallace P, Kadin ME. Evaluation of splenectomy in large granular lymphocyte leukaemia. *Br J Haematol.* 1987;67(2):135-140.

In: Neutropenia
Editors: M. Akhtari et al.
ISBN: 978-1-63482-105-6

Chapter 4

Chemotherapy-Induced Neutropenia: Determinants, Consequences and Prevention

***Vijaya Raj Bhatt*[1]*, Rajesh Shrestha*[2]*, Srujitha Murukutla*[3]*, Muniba Naqi*[3] *and Mojtaba Akhtari*[4]**

[1]University of Nebraska Medical Center,
Nebraska Medical Center, Omaha, NE, US
[2]Memorial Hospital of Rhode Island, Department of Internal Medicine,
Pawtucket, RI, US
[3]Staten Island University Hospital, Department of Internal Medicine,
Staten Island, NY, US
[4]Jane Anne Nohl Division of Hematology and Center for the Study of
Blood Diseases, University of Southern California (USC)/
Norris Cancer Center, USC University Hospital,
Keck Medical Center of USC, Los Angeles, CA, US

Introduction

For all practical purposes, neutropenia is defined as the absolute neutrophil count (ANC) of $< 1.5\times10^9$/L [1]. National Cancer Institute Common Toxicity Criteria for Adverse Events v3.0, the most common scale used for grading the severity of toxicity, divides treatment-related neutropenia into four grades according to the ANC: grade 1: ANC <lower limit of normal

to 1.5×10^9/L; grade 2: ANC $\geq$1.0 to < 1.5×10^9/L; grade 3: ANC $\geq$0.5 to < 1×10^9/L; and grade 4: ANC less than 0.5×10^9/L [2]. Acquired neutropenia is more common than congenital, frequently related to drug toxicity, and chemotherapeutic agents are among the most common causes [3]. The odds of neutropenia (or thrombocytopenia) and consequent complications is 14.6 times higher in patients undergoing chemotherapy than other patients [4]. Furthermore, chemotherapy-induced neutropenia (CIN) (ANC < 1×10^9/L) has been reported in 40% and severe CIN (ANC < 0.5×10^9/L) in 26% of cancer patients in a large prospective nationwide registry-based study [5]. Myelosuppressive regimens which were previously recommended for advanced or metastatic diseases, are more frequently used as neoadjuvant or adjuvant therapy in treating early-stage lung, colorectal and breast cancers [6]. Increased usage of myelosuppressive therapy will more likely lead to an escalated risk of CIN in the absence of preventive measures.

Simplified Model of Myelosuppression

Bone marrow hematopoietic cells are in various differentiation phases and can functionally be divided into three hypothetical compartments: proliferative, transit, and circulating compartments. Proliferative compartment harbors pluripotent stem cells and progenitor cells. Pluripotent stem cells are mitotically quiescent but have self-renewal capacity, whereas progenitor cells have extensive proliferation capacity but limited self-renewal capability. The progenitor cells undergo maturation through various stages in transit compartment and get delivered into circulating compartment as mature blood cells. Generation of new cells in proliferative compartment depends on both proliferation rate constant which determines the rate of cell division, and the number of dividing cells. Growth factors, cytokines, and a feedback mechanism from circulating cells affect cell division rate. From the transit compartment, cells move to circulation compartment where they ultimately die and degrade. In a normal healthy state, rate of proliferation, transit time, and circulating cells degradation is constant, and maintains hematopoietic cells balance in different compartments [7, 8]. In myelosuppression, growth factors are released and not only stimulate proliferating cells division in the marrow but also reduce the time at which mature cells reach the circulation [8].

Chemotherapeutic agents may reduce cell proliferation rate or induce cell death in bone marrow resulting into temporary marrow failure. Since the proliferation rate lags behind, the lost cells will not replenish, and eventually cytopenia occurs. Although chemotherapy may destroy in transit as well as circulating compartment hematopoietic cells, proliferating cells are generally more susceptible. Thus, marrow is significantly damaged before any change in peripheral blood count can be seen. In fact, rate of particular cytopenia development is determined by life blood cells span in circulation. Considering neutrophil's short life span of about ten hours, neutropenia secondary to chemotherapy-induced marrow failure occurs more rapidly compared to thrombocytopenia and anemia [7-9]. It takes 5 to 10 days after chemotherapy to reach ANC nadir in majority of patient [10].

Determinants and Prediction Models

Several factors including patient's characteristics, underlying disease and chemotherapy regimen determine probability of myelosuppression and CIN (table 1).

Table 1. Major determinants of chemotherapy-induced neutropenia

Patient Characteristics	Chemotherapy Regimen	Disease related factors
Advanced age: low marrow cellularity and delayed recovery [15, 67-69] *Poor performance status* [70] *Nutritional status*: Level of albumin determines the drug-binding [9], and the negative nitrogen balance is associated with low chemotherapy tolerance [71]. *Bone marrow compromise* (prior chemotherapy or radiation, or marrow infiltration) [9] *Pre-treatment laboratory tests*: White cell count, monocyte count [72], lymphocyte count [15], first-cycle nadir in white cell count [25, 26], pretreatment hemoglobin levels [71]. *Liver and kidney dysfunction, effusion or ascites* (compartmentalization of drugs leading to slow and prolonged release into the circulation) and *drug handling* (compliance, drug absorption, drug interaction) [9]	*Specific drugs(s), combination, and the number of drugs used* [11, 12, 73] *Dose Intensity* [70] *Combination with radiotherapy* [74] *Prophylactic use of colony stimulating factor* [75]	*Tumor type*: Greater in hematological malignancies [13] *Advanced disease* [74]

Among all of these factors, chemotherapy regimen plays a major role. Chemotherapeutic agents vary in their degree of myelotoxicity [11, 12]. Phase-specific agents such as methotrexate (S), bleomycin (G_2), and vincristine (M) cause early myelosuppression but marrow recovery also occurs rapidly. Phase non-specific but cell-cycle specific drugs such as anthracyclines, which are active during mitotic cycle lead to early marrow suppression the same as phase-specific agents but recovery takes comparatively longer. Cell-cycle non-specific agents such as nitrosoureas and busulfan may cause delayed and prolonged marrow suppression [7, 9]. Hematologic effect is more complex after repeated doses and regimen consisting of combination of cell-cycle specific and non-specific drugs. These effects also depend on the intensity of therapy to achieve remission or cure of the disease. In acute leukemia, drug dosages are formulated to produce a transient aplasia whereas chemotherapeutic regimen is tailored to prevent the occurrence of cytopenia in other types of malignancies [9].

Table 2. Individual scores of chemotherapeutic agents based on risk of neutropenia

Score	Chemotherapy Agents
0	Asparaginase, Bleomycin, Rituximab, Methotrexate + leucovorin,* Imatinib, Thalidomide, All trans retinoic acid (tretinoin), Bortezomib, Vincristine, Alemtuzumab
1	6-Thioguanine, 5-Fluorouracil, Cisplatin, Fludarabine,* Gemcitabine,* Chlorambucil, Vindesine,* Vinorelbine, Thiotepa, Hydroxyurea
2	Actinomycin D, Busulfan,* Carmustine,* Dacarbazine, Fludarabine,* Gemcitabine,* Mechlorethamine, Melphalan ($\leq$70 mg/m^2), Methotrexate,* Mitomycin C, Mitoxantrone, Mercaptopurine, Procabazine, Raltitrexed, Temozolomide, Vinblastine, Vindesine*
3	Cladribine, Adriamycin ($\leq$90 mg/m^2), Pemetrexed, Amsacrine, Bendamustine, Carboplatin, Cyclophosphamide ($\leq$1g/m^2), Cytarabine ($\leq$2g/m^2), Daunorubicin, Epirubicin, Etoposide ($\leq$100mg/m^2), Idarubicin,* Ifosfamide ($\leq$9g/m^2), Oxaliplatin, Teniposide
4	Adriamycin (>90 mg/m^2), Irinotecan, Topotecan, Busulfan,* Carmustine,*High dose Cisplatin, Cyclophosphamide (>1g/m^2), Cytarabine (>2g/m^2), Paclitaxel, Docetaxel, Etoposide (>100mg/m^2), Gemtuzumab, Idarubicin,* Ifosfamide (>9g/m^2), Melphalan (>70 mg/m^2)

* Different scores have been given to these agents in references [11] and [12].

In a retrospective analysis of 203, the possibility of predicting CIN duration based on the chemotherapy-specific risk factors was assessed [12].

Based on cytotoxicity and risk of inducing neutropenia, a simple score (0-4) was given to each chemotherapeutic agent (table 2), and two groups of high and low score was made. In this scoring system, a high score (≥ 8) was associated with 2 more additional days of CIN compared to a low score (<8) [12]. In a prospective study, 8 different factors were used as inclusion criteria for 266 hematological cancers, and patients were followed during 1053 chemotherapy cycles for febrile neutropenia (FN). This study showed that chemotherapy's score was the most important, and underlying disease was the second most important risk factors for developing FN; this makes aggressive chemotherapy regimen the main predictor of FN. This study provided a model with 13 variables and a total score of 35; higher score predicted greater risk of FN (table 3) [11].

Table 3. Baseline model for febrile neutropenia and weight score of the components

Items	Weight
Very aggressive Chemotherapy Regimen (score ≥3)	6
Acute myelogenous leukemia	7
Chronic myelogenous leukemia	9
Acute lymphocytic leukemia	6
Lymphoma and Hodgkin's disease	3
First cycle of a treatment line and baseline hemoglobin dosage <12 g/dl	8
First cycle of a treatment line and baseline hemoglobin dosage of ≥ 12 g/dl	7
Other cycles and baseline hemoglobin dosage <10 g/dl	7
Other cycles and baseline hemoglobin dosage ≥ 10 g/dl and <12 g/dl	6
Baseline monocyte count <150/μL	2
Bone marrow involvement	3
Body surface ≤ 2 m^2	3
Stem-cell transplantation	4
Total score	35

Consequences

CIN is one of the major dose limiting and life-threatening toxicities of chemotherapy and has several different implications: it increases morbidity and mortality, determines subsequent chemotherapy course and increases health care cost.

Morbidity and Mortality

CIN is the leading cause of hospitalization in cancer patients and can result in FN. Complications of CIN include life-threatening infection such as invasive fungal infection, pneumonia, gram negative sepsis and death. It has been shown that approximately 7-22% of cancer patients who are treated with chemotherapy require hospitalization for CIN [4]. National incidence rate of hospitalization for CIN is estimated to be 7.83 cases per 1000 cancer patients, and hematological malignancies, particularly leukemia have higher hospitalization rate [13]. Rate of FN depends on several factors including aggressiveness of chemotherapy regimen, and is less than 5% to more than 50% [14]. FN can increase mortality up to 10-20% of hospitalized patients [15-19]. Indeed, average morbidity and mortality rates are higher for patients with hematological malignancies than for those with solid tumors [20].

FN patients have different range of complications, and it is important to distinguish high-risk from low-risk patients. Several indicators have been used to make this distinction but one of the most widely used scoring systems is Multinational Association for Supportive Care in Cancer (MASCC) scoring system (Table 4). Positive predictive value of MASCC scoring system is as high as 91%, with specificity of 68% and sensitivity of 71%, and helps to identify patients at low risk complications (score $\geq$ 21 out of the maximum of 26) [21]. This scoring system helps to predict which patients can be treated as an outpatient. Besides MASCC risk index score less than 21 which is associated with unfavorable outcome, other high risk categories are patients with uncontrolled cancer, concurrent co-morbidities, and certain conditions such as tachypnea, thrombocytopenia, increased C-reactive protein and anticipated prolonged CIN [22, 23].

Table 4. Multinational Association for Supportive Care in Cancer scoring system [21]

Risk Factor	Points
Burden of illness: no or mild symptoms	5
No hypotension	5
No chronic obstructive pulmonary disease	4
Solid tumor and no previous fungal infection	4
No dehydration	3
Burden of illness: moderate symptoms	3
Outpatient status	3
Age <60 year	2

Impact on Subsequent Therapy

Treatment delay, dose reduction and permanent therapy discontinuation are some of CIN complications [24-28]. In a retrospective study, 50 patients with different types of solid tumors were randomly assessed for impact of neutropenia. The study revealed that 30% of patients had dose delay and 20% of patients had dose reduction secondary to CIN. Furthermore, relative dose intensity (RDI) in patients with or without CIN was 81% versus 92% respectively [28]. These consequences can potentially compromise survival outcome in patients receiving curative treatment [29-32]. In fact, even moderate dose reduction has negative impact on survival [29, 30, 33]. In many cancers such as diffuse large B-cell lymphoma [33] and node-positive breast cancer [30], dose reduction below 85-90% of optimal dose results in significantly poorer overall survival.

Economic Burden

Management of CIN imposes huge direct and indirect healthcare cost. In US, the cost of CIN may reach up to approximately 3,000 US dollars per outpatient episode and approximately 50,000 US dollars (both in 2006 value) per FN hospitalization. Compared to solid tumors, cost is even 2-3 times higher for patients with hematological malignancies especially leukemias. Cost is, however, much lower in other countries [4]. A study of FN admissions in 115 US hospitals based on University Health System Consortium hospitalization database showed that FN hospitalization resulted in an estimated cost of more than 1 billion over a 6-year interval [19]. In addition to cost for direct care, there are CIN- related indirect costs including patient work loss, caregiver work loss, paid care giver as well as cost of transportation and child care [15].

Quality of Life

CIN patients have fatigue and lack of energy, which is not related to hemoglobin level. Furthermore, CIN is associated with increased anxiety, social isolation and functional decline. FN, hospitalization and delay in chemotherapy have also been shown to worsen the stress. However, there is no biological explanation for psychological findings [15].

Prevention of CIN

Here, we describe several approaches to prevent CIN.

Modifications in Chemotherapy

Chemotherapy should be started after a careful assessment of risk and benefits. Chemotherapy should be avoided in high risk patients; such patients may be frail elderly patients with poor performance and multiple comorbidities. Furthermore, chemotherapy regimen with acceptable efficacy and lower risk of CIN is preferred whenever feasible [34]. According to American Society of Clinical Oncology (ASCO) improving quality of life or survival justifies using chemotherapy [35]. Therefore, in those patients who are receiving chemotherapy without curative extent, an appropriate dose modification is reasonable to reduce serious complications including risk of FN. However, as discussed above, dose reduction as a mean to prevent CIN may reduce survival. Although dose reduction is a common practice, it should be avoided as much as possible in curative intent chemotherapy.

Prophylactic Antibiotic Therapy

Prophylactic antibiotics are another modality to manage CIN complications such as FN. Cochrane database reviewed 95 randomized controlled clinical trials of antibiotic prophylaxis in CIN patients which performed between 1973 and 2004. This meta-analysis revealed that comparing with placebo or simply no treatment, prophylactic antibiotics significantly decreased all-cause mortality in CIN patients. However, all of these trials showed that prophylactic antibiotic therapy in CIN patients increases risk of resistant infections. Quinolones are one of the popular broad spectrum antibiotics that were assessed in 52 trials for prophylaxis in patients with CIN. All-cause mortality, microbiologically and clinically-documented infections, gram negative and gram positive infections, fever, and infection-related mortality were decreased by fluoroquinolone prophylaxis. The incidence of harboring resistance or outbreaks of resistant bacteria due to fluoroquinolone prophylaxis was much lower than trimethoprim-sulfamethoxazole. The addition of gram-positive antibiotics to fluoroquinolone resulted in decrease in microbiologically documented infections, bacteremia and gram-positive bacteremia without any mortality benefit. Hematological malignancies were studied in most of these clinical trials. The methodological quality of these trials was not the same which was another limitation of these studies. This meta-analysis demonstrated that prophylactic antibiotic therapy in neutropenic patients, preferably with fluoroquinolone reduces mortality and especially should be considered in a subset of hematological cancer patients with neutropenia [36]. Prophylactic levofloxacin was used in two prospective, double-blind, randomized control trials of patients with acute leukemia, solid tumors or lymphoma and expected CIN after myelosuppressive chemotherapy. In both studies, prophylactic levofloxacin significantly reduced incidence of FN, clinically and microbiologically documented infection, hospitalization and length of stay [37, 38]. Thus, it is rational to start prophylactic fluoroquinolones in high-risk neutropenic patients, especially those with hematological malignancies who are undergoing myelosuppressive therapy. A meta-analysis of 64 randomized controlled clinical trial of prophylactic antifungal therapy in cancer patients has been found that prophylactic antifungal therapy reduced all-cause mortality as well as fungal-related mortality and documented invasive fungal infection (IFI) in patients with allogeneic stem cell transplant (allo-SCT). However, the difference of fungal-related mortality and documented IFI in acute leukemia patients was borderline significant [39]. In a retrospective study of 86 recipients of allogeneic hematopoietic stem cell transplantation, prophylactic, long-term low-dose acyclovir significantly decreased varicella zoster virus reactivation [40]. In a double blind, placebo controlled study of 93 cytomegalovirus (CMV) seropositive allograft bone marrow transplant recipients, CMV infection dropped from 45% in placebo group to 3% in prophylactic ganciclovir recipients in the first one hundred days [41]. Prophylactic acyclovir has been assessed in a double blind, placebo-controlled study on 20 seropositive herpes simplex virus (HSV) bone marrow transplant recipients. Seven out of 10 control patients developed culture positive HSV lesions while acyclovir recipients were symptom free [42]. Prophylactic antifungal and antiviral therapy should be utilized for high risk CIN patients such as acute leukemia and bone marrow transplant recipients.

National Comprehensive Cancer Network (NCCN) and Infectious Diseases Society of America (IDSA) have recently updated guidelines of prophylactic antibiotic in CIN separately [43, 44]. NCCN guideline is somewhat more comprehensive and elaborates on the antimicrobial prophylaxis in several chemotherapy regimens as well as oncological conditions. According to NCCN guidelines, antimicrobial prophylaxis is not indicated for low risk patients (patients with solid tumors receiving standard chemotherapy regimens and patients with anticipated duration of CIN <7 days). Unlike IDSA, NCCN has an intermediate risk category which includes patients with anticipated CIN of 7 to 10 days, patients with lymphoma, multiple myeloma, chronic lymphocytic leukemia, autologous SCT (auto-SCT) recipients, and patients on purine analog therapy. Fluoroquinolones are a good choice for intermediate risk patients. For autologous hematopoietic stem cell recipients and neutropenic patients, prophylactic antivirals should be started and continued for at least 30 days post-transplant. Antifungals should be considered for intermediate patients in neutropenic phase and autologous SCT with anticipated mucositis [44]. Allo-SCT recipients or post allo-SCT graft-versus-host-disease (GVHD) patients, patients who are taking alemtuzumab, acute leukemia patients on induction and consolidation therapy, and patients with expected neutropenia more than 10 days are considered high risk, and prophylactic antibacterials such as fluoroquinolone are indicated. Prophylactic antivirals are indicated in neutropenic phase of high risk patients and should be continued for at least 30 days post-transplant. Acute lymphocytic leukemia (ALL) patients, acute myeloid leukemia (AML)/myelodysplatic syndrome (MDS) patients with neutropenia, allo-SCT recipients, and patients with significant GVHD should receive prophylactic antifungals. A proteasome inhibitor, bortezomib, increases risk of varicella zoster reactivation in patients with history of chicken pox, and prophylactic antiviral therapy with acyclovir, valacyclovir or famciclovir is indicated. HSV prophylaxis should be considered for chronic lymphocytic leukemia (CLL) patients receiving CD52 monoclonal antibody alemtuzumab, prolonged neutropenia in hematologic malignancy patients or patients who are receiving high dose corticosteroids or T-cell depleting agents such as fludarabine. Patients undergoing alemtuzumab treatment require monitoring for cytomegalovirus infection or reactivation once a week for CMV antigen or polymerase chain reaction testing till at least 2 months after alemtuzumab therapy. CMV monitoring and pre-emptive therapy should be utilized in CMV seropositive allo-SCT recipients, particularly if either donor or recipient is positive for CMV. It should be emphasized that some antiviral agents are bone marrow suppressor and should be used cautiously in select patients. Pneumocystis jiroveci prophylaxis is recommended for allo-SCT recipients, ALL, alemtuzumab therapy, purine analog therapy, as well as concurrent temozolomide and radiation therapy till lymphocytopenia resolved.

Use of Granulocyte Colony-Stimulating Factor

Granulocyte colony-stimulating factors (G-CSF) may decrease FN incidence, FN-related hospitalization, use of intravenous antibiotics, infection-related mortality and need for chemotherapy dose modification [45-48]. A meta-analysis of 17 randomized control trials (n=3493) showed that comparing to placebo, primary prophylactic G-CSF reduces risk of FN, infection-related mortality and all-cause mortality during chemotherapy in adult patients with solid tumor and malignant lymphoma. Furthermore, relative dose intensity (RDI) of chemotherapy was significantly higher with G-CSF. However, G-CSF was associated with more musculoskeletal pain [49]. Although economic analysis have shown that primary prophylaxis of G-CSF is cost-effective, secondary prophylaxis by antibiotics is the least expensive strategy and antibiotics are the mainstay of treatment in FN patients [50]. Similarly, another meta-analysis of 13 randomized control trials comparing CSFs plus antibiotics versus antibiotics alone in FN (n=1518) showed that use of G-CSF for chemotherapy-induced FN reduces length of stay and neutrophil recovery time. In this meta-analysis, use of CSFs was associated with a marginally significant reduction in infection-related mortality but overall mortality did not change [47]. Although there is some role for G-CSF in the management of established FN, concerns have been raised about the association between AML/MDS and use of G-CSF. A meta-analysis of 25 randomized control trials (n=12,804) was done to evaluate use of G-CSF and risk of AML or MDS in patients who are receiving chemotherapy. This meta-analysis demonstrated that use of G-CSF increased RDI and risk of AML/MDS but decreased all-cause mortality. Although no significant association was noticed between RDI and relative risk of AML/MDS after G-CSF use, comparing to controls, there was significant association between relative and absolute increase in RDI, and G-CSF use reduced mortality [51].

Filgrastim and pegfilgrastim are the most commonly used G-CSF. Studies comparing effectiveness of two G-CSFs have shown that pegfilgrastim is more effective on reducing risk of FN and hospitalization for neutropenic complications than filgrastim [46, 52-54]. In a retrospective cohort study, effect of prophylactic pegfilgrastim or filgrastim on risk of hospitalization due to neutropenic complications in patients with solid tumors was evaluated. Compared to pegfilgrastim, filgrastim was associated with one third higher risk of hospitalization for neutropenic complications [55]. Combination of pegfilgrastim and ciprofloxacin may be even more effective. Another study has shown that risk of FN was decreased to 7% when pegfilgrastim was used alone and to 5% when pegfilgrastim was combined with ciprofloxacin. This was significantly lower than risk of FN with filgrastim (18%) or ciprofloxacin alone (22%). Furthermore, combination of pegfilgrastim and ciprofloxacin, compared to pegfilgrastim alone, was significantly more effective in preventing first cycle FN (0% vs 2%) [54]. Although prophylactic use of pegfilgrastim is expensive, it has been shown to be cost-effective [54, 56-59] and even cost saving [58].

Independent guidelines for use of CSF has been published by ASCO, NCCN, IDSA, European Society for Medical Oncology and European Organization for Research and Treatment of Cancer [14, 34, 43, 44, 60, 61]. These guidelines are fairly consistent and provide following recommendations. Primary prophylactic G-CSF is recommended in any chemotherapy regimen associated with risk of FN ≥20%. If risk of FN is 10%-20%, G-CSF should be considered for patients with following characteristics which predispose them to increased risk of FN or increased complications of FN: age >65, poor performance or nutritional status, previous history of FN, extensive prior treatment, advanced-stage cancer, bone marrow infiltration by cancer with subsequent cytopenias, presence of open-wounds, recent surgery or active infections and other serious co-morbidities such as liver or kidney dysfunction. For patients undergoing concomitant chemotherapy and radiation, particularly mediastinal radiation and when risk of FN is <10%, G-CSF is not recommended. When indicated, daily G-CSF or filgrastim should be initiated 24-72 hours after completion of chemotherapy and continued until ANC is >2-3000/μL. Pegylated G-CSF (pegfilgrastim) dose is given only once. Administration of G-CSF before, during or 24 hours after chemotherapy should be avoided.

A new G-CSF, tbo-filgrastim (XM02) has been FDA approved for use in non-myeloid malignancy patients receiving chemotherapy associated with significant risk of FN (www.fda.gov). Approval was based on results of trials in patients with breast cancer [62], lung cancer [63] and non-Hodgkin lymphoma [64] which showed tbo-filgrastim is as effective as filgrastim in reducing FN or duration of severe CIN. Several ongoing studies are trying to develop and evaluate other G-CSFs. In particular, studies are evaluating safety and efficacy of novel pegylated G-CSFs in non-small cell lung cancer (ClinicalTrials.gov ID NCT01560195), and breast cancer (NCT00501332, NCT01569087, NCT01674855 and NCT01328938) patients who are receiving myelosuppressive chemotherapy. Studies are also looking into pharmacokinetics and pharmacodynamics of novel pegylated G-CSFs in healthy male volunteers (NCT00969826). Recently, new compounds are also being synthesized in an attempt to enhance efficacy of G-CSF, simplify its production or improve its stability and pharmacokinetics [65, 66]. Development of more effective G-CSFs will improve treatment outcome in CIN patients.

Conclusion

CIN is one of the major dose limiting and life-threatening toxicities of chemotherapy, and has multifaceted implications: it increases morbidity and mortality, determines courses of subsequent chemotherapy, and increases health care cost. Use of CSF in a timely manner during chemotherapy and prophylactic antimicrobials in intermediate to high risk patients can significantly decrease risk of FN and its complications and allow completion of planned chemotherapy.

References

[1] Haddy, TB; Rana, SR; Castro, O. Benign ethnic neutropenia: what is a normal absolute neutrophil count? *J Lab Clin Med*. 1999 Jan, 133(1),15-22.

[2] Common Terminology Criteria for Adverse Events v3.0 (CTCAE)2006: Available from:http://ctep.cancer.gov/protocolDevelopment/ electronic_ applications/docs/ ctcaev3.pdf.

[3] Munshi, HG; Montgomery, RB. Severe neutropenia: a diagnostic approach. *West J Med*. 2000 Apr, 172(4), 248-52.

[4] Liou, SY; Stephens, JM; Carpiuc, KT; Feng, W; Botteman, MF; Hay, JW. Economic burden of haematological adverse effects in cancer patients: a systematic review. *Clin Drug Investig*. 2007, 27(6), 381-96.

[5] Wolff, DA; Crawford, J; Dale, DC; Poniewierski, MS; Lyman, GH. Risk of neutropenic complications based on a prospective nationwide registry of cancer patients initiating systematic chemotherapy. *J Clin Oncol*. 2004, 22, No 14S (July 15 Supplement), Abstract: 6125.

[6] Smith, RE. Trends in recommendations for myelosuppressive chemotherapy for the treatment of solid tumors. J *Natl Compr Canc Netw*. 2006 Aug, 4(7), 649-58.

[7] Kim, SK; Demetri, GD., Chemotherapy and neutropenia. *Hematol Oncol Clin North Am*. 1996 Apr, 10(2), 377-95.

[8] Friberg, LE; Henningsson, A; Maas, H; Nguyen, L; Karlsson, MO. Model of chemotherapy-induced myelosuppression with parameter consistency across drugs. *J Clin Oncol*. 2002 Dec 15, 20(24), 4713-21.

[9] Bodensteiner, DC; Doolittle, GC. Adverse haematological complications of anticancer drugs. Clinical presentation, management and avoidance. *Drug Saf*. 1993 Mar, 8(3), 213-24.

[10] Capo, G; Waltzman, R. Managing hematologic toxicities. *J Support Oncol*. 2004 Jan-Feb, 2(1), 65-79.

[11] Moreau, M; Klastersky, J; Schwarzbold, A; Muanza, F; Georgala, A; Aoun, M; et al. A general chemotherapy myelotoxicity score to predict febrile neutropenia in hematological malignancies. *Ann Oncol*. 2009 Mar, 20(3), 513-9.

[12] Lalami, Y; Paesmans, M; Muanza, F; Barette, M; Plehiers, B; Dubreucq, L; et al. Can we predict the duration of chemotherapy-induced neutropenia in febrile neutropenic patients, focusing on regimen-specific risk factors? A retrospective analysis. *Ann Oncol*. 2006 Mar, 17(3), 507-14.

[13] Caggiano, V; Weiss, RV; Rickert, TS; Linde-Zwirble, WT. Incidence, cost, and mortality of neutropenia hospitalization associated with chemotherapy. *Cancer*. 2005 May 1, 103(9), 1916-24.

[14] Aapro, MS; Bohlius, J; Cameron, DA; Dal, Lago, L; Donnelly, JP; Kearney, N; et al. 2010 update of EORTC guidelines for the use of granulocyte-colony stimulating factor to reduce the incidence of chemotherapy-induced febrile neutropenia in adult patients with lymphoproliferative disorders and solid tumours. *Eur J Cancer*. 2011 Jan, 47(1), 8-32.

[15] Daniel, D; Crawford, J. Myelotoxicity from chemotherapy. *Semin Oncol*. 2006 Feb, 33(1), 74-85.

[16] Talcott, JA; Siegel, RD; Finberg, R; Goldman, L. Risk assessment in cancer patients with fever and neutropenia: a prospective, two-center validation of a prediction rule. *J Clin Oncol*. 1992 Feb, 10(2), 316-22.

[17] Pizzo, PA; Hathorn, JW; Hiemenz, J; Browne, M; Commers, J; Cotton, D; et al. A randomized trial comparing ceftazidime alone with combination antibiotic therapy in cancer patients with fever and neutropenia. *N Engl J Med*. 1986 Aug 28, 315(9), 552-8.

[18] Schimpff, SC; Gaya, H; Klastersky, J; Tattersall, MH; Zinner, SH. Three antibiotic regimens in the treatment of infection in febrile granulocytopenic patients with cancer. The EORTC international antimicrobial therapy project group. *J Infect Dis*. 1978 Jan, 137(1), 14-29.

[19] Kuderer, NM; Dale, DC; Crawford, J; Cosler, LE; Lyman, GH. Mortality, morbidity, and cost associated with febrile neutropenia in adult cancer patients. *Cancer*. 2006 May 15, 106(10), 2258-66.

[20] Marti, FM; Cullen, MH; Roila, F. Management of febrile neutropenia: ESMO clinical recommendations. *Ann Oncol*. 2009 May, 20 Suppl 4, 166-9.

[21] Klastersky, J; Paesmans, M; Rubenstein, EB; Boyer, M; Elting, L; Feld, R; et al. The Multinational Association for Supportive Care in Cancer risk index: A multinational scoring system for identifying low-risk febrile neutropenic cancer patients. *J Clin Oncol*. 2000 Aug, 18(16), 3038-51.

[22] Talcott, JA; Finberg, R; Mayer, RJ; Goldman, L. The medical course of cancer patients with fever and neutropenia. Clinical identification of a low-risk subgroup at presentation. *Arch Intern Med*. 1988 Dec, 148(12), 2561-8.

[23] Ahn, S; Lee, YS; Chun, YH; Kwon, IH; Kim, W; Lim, KS; et al. Predictive factors of poor prognosis in cancer patients with chemotherapy-induced febrile neutropenia. *Support Care Cancer*. 2011 Aug, 19 (8), 1151-8.

[24] Chrischilles, EA; Link, BK; Scott, SD; Delgado, DJ; Fridman, M. Factors associated with early termination of CHOP therapy and the impact on survival among patients with chemosensitive intermediate-grade non-Hodgkin's lymphoma. *Cancer Control*. 2003 Sep-Oct, 10(5), 396-403.

[25] Silber, JH; Fridman, M; DiPaola, RS; Erder, MH; Pauly, MV; Fox, KR. First-cycle blood counts and subsequent neutropenia, dose reduction, or delay in early-stage breast cancer therapy. *J Clin Oncol*. 1998 Jul, 16(7), 2392-400.

[26] Savvides, P; Terrin, N; Erban, J; Selker, HP. Development and validation of a patient-specific predictive instrument for the need for dose reduction in chemotherapy for breast cancer: a potential decision aid for the use of myeloid growth factors. *Support Care Cancer*. 2003 May, 11(5), 313-20.

[27] Link, BK; Budd, GT; Scott, S; Dickman, E; Paul, D; Lawless, G; et al. Delivering adjuvant chemotherapy to women with early-stage breast carcinoma: current patterns of care. *Cancer*. 2001 Sep 15, 92(6), 1354-67.

[28] Khan, S; Dhadda, A; Fyfe, D; Sundar, S. Impact of neutropenia on delivering planned chemotherapy for solid tumours. *Eur J Cancer Care (Engl)*. 2008 Jan, 17(1), 19-25.

[29] Kwak, LW; Halpern, J; Olshen, RA; Horning, SJ. Prognostic significance of actual dose intensity in diffuse large-cell lymphoma: results of a tree-structured survival analysis. *J Clin Oncol*. 1990 Jun, 8(6), 963-77.

[30] Bonadonna, G; Valagussa, P; Moliterni, A; Zambetti, M; Brambilla, C. Adjuvant cyclophosphamide, methotrexate, and fluorouracil in node-positive breast cancer: the results of 20 years of follow-up. *N Engl J Med*. 1995 Apr 6, 332(14), 901-6.

[31] Ardizzoni, A; Favaretto, A; Boni, L; Baldini, E; Castiglioni, F; Antonelli, P; et al. Platinum-etoposide chemotherapy in elderly patients with small-cell lung cancer: results of a randomized multicenter phase II study assessing attenuated-dose or full-dose with lenograstim prophylaxis--a Forza Operativa Nazionale Italiana Carcinoma

Polmonare and Gruppo Studio Tumori Polmonari Veneto (FONICAP-GSTPV) study. *J Clin Oncol.* 2005 Jan 20, 23(3), 569-75.

[32] Budman, DR; Berry, DA; Cirrincione, CT; Henderson, IC; Wood, WC; Weiss, RB; et al. Dose and dose intensity as determinants of outcome in the adjuvant treatment of breast cancer. The Cancer and Leukemia Group B. *J Natl Cancer Inst.* 1998 Aug 19, 90(16), 1205-11.

[33] Bosly, A; Bron, D; Van, Hoof, A; De, Bock, R; Berneman, Z; Ferrant, A; et al. Achievement of optimal average relative dose intensity and correlation with survival in diffuse large B-cell lymphoma patients treated with CHOP. *Ann Hematol.* 2008 Apr, 87(4), 277-83.

[34] Smith, TJ; Khatcheressian, J; Lyman, GH; Ozer, H; Armitage, JO; Balducci, L; et al. 2006 update of recommendations for the use of white blood cell growth factors: an evidence-based clinical practice guideline. *J Clin Oncol.* 2006 Jul 1, 24(19), 3187-205.

[35] Outcomes of cancer treatment for technology assessment and cancer treatment guidelines. American Society of Clinical Oncology. *J Clin Oncol.* 1996 Feb, 14(2), 671-9.

[36] Gafter-Gvili, A; Fraser, A; Paul, M; Leibovici, L. Meta-analysis: antibiotic prophylaxis reduces mortality in neutropenic patients. *Ann Intern Med.* 2005 Jun 21, 142(12 Pt 1), 979-95.

[37] Bucaneve, G; Micozzi, A; Menichetti, F; Martino, P; Dionisi, MS; Martinelli, G; et al. Levofloxacin to prevent bacterial infection in patients with cancer and neutropenia. *N Engl J Med.* 2005 Sep 8, 353(10), 977-87.

[38] Cullen, M; Steven, N; Billingham, L; Gaunt, C; Hastings, M; Simmonds, P; et al. Antibacterial prophylaxis after chemotherapy for solid tumors and lymphomas. *N Engl J Med.* 2005 Sep 8, 353(10), 988-98.

[39] Robenshtok, E; Gafter-Gvili, A; Goldberg, E; Weinberger, M; Yeshurun, M; Leibovici, L; et al. Antifungal prophylaxis in cancer patients after chemotherapy or hematopoietic stem-cell transplantation: systematic review and meta-analysis. *J Clin Oncol.* 2007 Dec 1, 25(34), 5471-89.

[40] Kanda, Y; Mineishi, S; Saito, T; Saito, A; Yamada, S; Ohnishi, M; et al. Long-term low-dose acyclovir against varicella-zoster virus reactivation after allogeneic hematopoietic stem cell transplantation. *Bone Marrow Transplant.* 2001 Oct, 28(7), 689-92.

[41] Goodrich, JM; Bowden, RA; Fisher, L; Keller, C; Schoch, G; Meyers, JD. Ganciclovir prophylaxis to prevent cytomegalovirus disease after

allogeneic marrow transplant. *Ann Intern Med*. 1993 Feb 1, 118(3), 173-8.

[42] Saral, R; Burns, WH; Laskin, OL; Santos, GW; Lietman, PS. Acyclovir prophylaxis of herpes-simplex-virus infections. *N Engl J Med*. 1981 Jul 9, 305(2), 63-7.

[43] Freifeld, AG; Bow, EJ; Sepkowitz, KA; Boeckh, MJ; Ito, JI; Mullen, CA; et al. Clinical practice guideline for the use of antimicrobial agents in neutropenic patients with cancer: 2010 update by the infectious diseases society of america. *Clin Infect Dis*. 2011 Feb 15, 52(4), e56-93.

[44] Baden, LR; Bensinger, W; Angarone, M; Casper, C; Dubberke, ER; Freifeld, AG; et al. Prevention and Treatment of Cancer-Related Infections. *Journal of the National Comprehensive Cancer Network*. 2012 November 1, 2012, 10(11), 1412-45.

[45] von, Minckwitz, G; Schwenkglenks, M; Skacel, T; Lyman, GH; Pousa, AL; Bacon, P; et al. Febrile neutropenia and related complications in breast cancer patients receiving pegfilgrastim primary prophylaxis versus current practice neutropaenia management: results from an integrated analysis. *Eur J Cancer*. 2009 Mar, 45(4), 608-17.

[46] Renwick, W; Pettengell, R; Green, M. Use of filgrastim and pegfilgrastim to support delivery of chemotherapy: twenty years of clinical experience. *BioDrugs*. 2009, 23(3), 175-86.

[47] Clark, OA; Lyman, GH; Castro, AA; Clark, LG; Djulbegovic, B. Colony-stimulating factors for chemotherapy-induced febrile neutropenia: a meta-analysis of randomized controlled trials. J Clin Oncol. 2005 Jun 20, 23(18), 4198-214.

[48] Cooper, KL; Madan, J; Whyte, S; Stevenson, MD; Akehurst, RL. Granulocyte colony-stimulating factors for febrile neutropenia prophylaxis following chemotherapy: systematic review and meta-analysis. *BMC Cancer*. 2011, 11, 404.

[49] Kuderer, NM; Dale, DC; Crawford, J; Lyman, GH. Impact of primary prophylaxis with granulocyte colony-stimulating factor on febrile neutropenia and mortality in adult cancer patients receiving chemotherapy: a systematic review. *J Clin Oncol*. 2007 Jul 20, 25(21), 3158-67.

[50] Dale, DC. Advances in the treatment of neutropenia. *Curr Opin Support Palliat Care*. 2009 Sep, 3(3), 207-12.

[51] Lyman, GH; Dale, DC; Wolff, DA; Culakova, E; Poniewierski, MS; Kuderer, NM; et al. Acute myeloid leukemia or myelodysplastic syndrome in randomized controlled clinical trials of cancer

chemotherapy with granulocyte colony-stimulating factor: a systematic review. *J Clin Oncol.* 2010 Jun 10, 28(17), 2914-24.

[52] Weycker, D; Malin, J; Barron, R; Edelsberg, J; Kartashov, A; Oster, G. Comparative effectiveness of filgrastim, pegfilgrastim, and sargramostim as prophylaxis against hospitalization for neutropenic complications in patients with cancer receiving chemotherapy. *Am J Clin Oncol.* 2012 Jun, 35(3), 267-74.

[53] Henk, HJ; Becker, L; Tan, H; Yu, J; Kavati, A; Naeim, A; et al. Comparative effectiveness of pegfilgrastim, filgrastim, and sargramostim prophylaxis for neutropenia-related hospitalization: two US retrospective claims analyses. *J Med Econ.* 2013, 16(1), 160-8.

[54] von, Minckwitz, G; Kummel, S; du, Bois, A; Eiermann, W; Eidtmann, H; Gerber, B; et al. Pegfilgrastim +/- ciprofloxacin for primary prophylaxis with TAC (docetaxel/ doxorubicin/ cyclophosphamide) chemotherapy for breast cancer. Results from the GEPARTRIO study. *Ann Oncol.* 2008 Feb, 19(2), 292-8.

[55] Weycker, D; Malin, J; Kim, J; Barron, R; Edelsberg, J; Kartashov, A; et al. Risk of hospitalization for neutropenic complications of chemotherapy in patients with primary solid tumors receiving pegfilgrastim or filgrastim prophylaxis: a retrospective cohort study. *Clin Ther.* 2009 May, 31(5), 1069-81.

[56] Almenar, D; Mayans, J; Juan, O; Bueno, JM; Lopez, JI; Frau, A; et al. Pegfilgrastim and daily granulocyte colony-stimulating factor: patterns of use and neutropenia-related outcomes in cancer patients in Spain--results of the LEARN Study. *Eur J Cancer Care (Engl).* 2009 May, 18(3), 280-6.

[57] Danova, M; Chiroli, S; Rosti, G; Doan, QV. Cost-effectiveness of pegfilgrastim versus six days of filgrastim for preventing febrile neutropenia in breast cancer patients. *Tumori.* 2009 Mar-Apr, 95(2), 219-26.

[58] Eldar-Lissai, A; Cosler, LE; Culakova, E; Lyman, GH. Economic analysis of prophylactic pegfilgrastim in adult cancer patients receiving chemotherapy. *Value Health.* 2008 Mar-Apr, 11(2), 172-9.

[59] Lyman, G; Lalla, A; Barron, R; Dubois, RW. Cost-effectiveness of pegfilgrastim versus 6-day filgrastim primary prophylaxis in patients with non-Hodgkin's lymphoma receiving CHOP-21 in United States. *Curr Med Res Opin.* 2009 Feb, 25(2), 401-11.

[60] Crawford, J; Allen, J; Armitage, J; Blayney, DW; Cataland, SR; Heaney, ML; et al. Myeloid Growth Factors. *Journal of the National Comprehensive Cancer Network*. 2011 August 1, 2011, 9(8), 914-32.

[61] Crawford, J; Caserta, C; Roila, F. Hematopoietic growth factors: ESMO recommendations for the applications. *Ann Oncol*. 2009 May, 20 Suppl 4, 162-5.

[62] del, Giglio, A; Eniu, A; Ganea-Motan, D; Topuzov, E; Lubenau, H. XM02 is superior to placebo and equivalent to Neupogen in reducing the duration of severe neutropenia and the incidence of febrile neutropenia in cycle 1 in breast cancer patients receiving docetaxel/doxorubicin chemotherapy. *BMC Cancer*. 2008, 8, 332.

[63] Gatzemeier, U; Ciuleanu, T; Dediu, M; Ganea-Motan, E; Lubenau, H; Del Giglio, A. XM02, the first biosimilar G-CSF, is safe and effective in reducing the duration of severe neutropenia and incidence of febrile neutropenia in patients with small cell or non-small cell lung cancer receiving platinum-based chemotherapy. *J Thorac Oncol*. 2009 Jun, 4(6), 736-40.

[64] Engert, A; Griskevicius, L; Zyuzgin, Y; Lubenau, H; del, Giglio, A. XM02, the first granulocyte colony-stimulating factor biosimilar, is safe and effective in reducing the duration of severe neutropenia and incidence of febrile neutropenia in patients with non-Hodgkin lymphoma receiving chemotherapy. *Leuk Lymphoma*. 2009 Mar, 50(3), 374-9.

[65] Natalello, A; Ami, D; Collini, M; D'Alfonso, L; Chirico, G; Tonon, G; et al. Biophysical characterization of Met-G-CSF: effects of different site-specific mono-pegylations on protein stability and aggregation. *PLoS One*. 2012, 7(8), e42511.

[66] Scaramuzza, S; Tonon, G; Olianas, A; Messana, I; Schrepfer, R; Orsini, G; et al. A new site-specific monoPEGylated filgrastim derivative prepared by enzymatic conjugation: Production and physicochemical characterization. *J Control Release*. 2012 Dec 28, 164(3), 355-63.

[67] Crawford, J; Dale, DC; Lyman, GH. Chemotherapy-induced neutropenia: risks, consequences, and new directions for its management. *Cancer*. 2004 Jan 15, 100(2), 228-37.

[68] Schouten, HC. Neutropenia management. *Ann Oncol*. 2006 Sep, 17 Suppl 10, x85-9.

[69] Khalil, F; Cualing, H; Cogburn, J; Miles, L. The criteria for bone marrow recovery post-myelosuppressive therapy for acute myelogenous leukemia: a quantitative study. *Arch Pathol Lab Med*. 2007 Aug, 131(8), 1281-9.

[70] Lyman, GH; Lyman, CH; Agboola, O. Risk models for predicting chemotherapy-induced neutropenia. *Oncologist*. 2005 Jun-Jul, 10(6), 427-37.

[71] Intragumtornchai, T; Sutheesophon, J; Sutcharitchan, P; Swasdikul, D. A predictive model for life-threatening neutropenia and febrile neutropenia after the first course of CHOP chemotherapy in patients with aggressive non-Hodgkin's lymphoma. *Leuk Lymphoma*. 2000 Apr, 37(3-4), 351-60.

[72] Kondo, M; Oshita, F; Kato, Y; Yamada, K; Nomura, I; Noda, K. Early monocytopenia after chemotherapy as a risk factor for neutropenia. Am *J Clin Oncol*. 1999 Feb, 22(1), 103-5.

[73] Lyman, GH; Kuderer, NM; Crawford, J; Wolff, DA; Culakova, E; Poniewierski, MS; et al. Prospective validation of a risk model for first cycle neutropenic complications in patients receiving cancer chemotherapy. *ASCO Meeting Abstracts*. 2006 June 16, 2006, 24(18_suppl), 8561.

[74] Leonard, R; Szucs, TD; Pettengell, R; Paridaens, R; Jackisch, C; Constenla, M; et al. Dose-limiting effects of neutropenic events in six European audits of adjuvant breast cancer chemotherapy. *J Clin Oncol*. 2004, 22, No 14S (July 15 Supplement), Abstract, 619.

[75] Dale, DC. Colony-stimulating factors for the management of neutropenia in cancer patients. *Drugs*. 2002, 62 Suppl 1, 1-15.

In: Neutropenia
Editors: M. Akhtari et al.
ISBN: 978-1-63482-105-6

Chapter 5

Mycobacterium tuberculosis and Non-tuberculous Mycobacterium Infections in Hematological Patients with Febrile Neutropenia

***Chien-Yuan Chen*[1]*, Ming-Shu Hsieh*[2] *and Wang-Huei Sheng*[1]**
[1]Departments of Internal Medicine and [2]Pathology,
National Taiwan University Hospital, Taipei, Taiwan

Introduction

Febrile neutropenia is one of the most serious complications in patients with hematological malignancies who received chemotherapy. Aerobic bacteria and fungi are the leading causative pathogens for febrile neutropenia. *Mycobacterium tuberculosis* (MTB) is a slow growing microbe that can cause clinical disease in both healthy and immunocompromised persons. Since *M. tuberculosis* is a rare pathogen causing clinical syndrome in developed countries and might mimic several common bacterial pathogens, misdiagnosis and delay treatment for *M. tuberculosis* diseases (tuberculosis) is not uncommon and might lead to grave prognosis. On the other hand, tuberculosis has shown resurgence in low endemic countries recently, a phenomenon that has been attributed to factors such as increased migration, advance of cancer chemotherapy agent and immunosuppressant, organ transplantation and the human immunodeficiency virus (HIV) epidemic. Therefore, tuberculosis and non-tuberculous mycobacteria (NTM) associated diseases could not be neglected among the patients with hematological malignancies in febrile neutropenia [1-5].

Table 1. Incidence of tuberculosis in different countries

Country or Area	Incidence (per 100000 population)		References
	general population	patients with hematological malignancy	
United States	3.4	61-457	[9, 12]
France	4.3 (4-4.6)		[15]
Germany	4.5 (3.9-5.1)		[15]
Japan	< 20		[13]
Brazil	42 (35-50)		[15]
Taiwan	74.6	120	[3, 10]
China	75 (66-85)		[15]
Russia	97 (82-114)		[15]
India	181 (163-199)		[15]
Indonesia	187 (155-222)		[15]
sub-Saharan Africa	> 260		[11]
South Africa	993 (819-1180)		[15]

Epidemiology

In southeastern Asia and sub-Saharan Africa, tuberculosis is a relatively common infectious disease. In general population, incidence of tuberculosis was 3.4 cases per 100,000 persons in United States [6], compared with 74.6 cases per 100, 000 persons in Taiwan [7], and over 260 cases per 100, 000 persons in sub-Saharan Africa [8]. The incidence of tuberculosis varied significantly according to country of birth [9], and is 61 per 100,000 persons in US-born patients with hematological malignancies, and 457 per 100,000 persons in non-US-born patients with hematological malignancies. Epidemiology of tuberculosis in different countries is listed in Table 1 [6-12].

Incidence of tuberculosis also varies significantly according to cancer type [9]. Patients with hematological malignancies have the higher risk to develop MTB and NTM associated infections than the patients with solid cancer. In the United States, foreign-born patients with underlying hematological malignancies had a tuberculosis rate 50-100 times higher than US-born patients, whereas US-born patients with solid cancers had similar prevalence of tuberculosis as that of US-born persons without cancer [9]. However, patients with hematological malignancies had 4-7 folds of risk of tuberculosis than the patients with solid cancer [9]. The estimated incidence of proved tuberculosis based on positive culture for MTB was 120 per 100,000 adult patients with hematological malignancies in Taiwan [3].

Epidemiology of NTM associated diseases in general population is relatively limited [13-18]. In England, incidence of NTM associated diseases increased from 0.9 per 100,000 population in 1995 to 2.9 per 100,000 in 2006 [13]. The median incidence rates of overall NTM associated diseases, *Mycobacterium avium-intracellulare* complex (MAC) and non-MAC diseases were 6.7, 4.5 and < 0.7 per 100,000 population in British Columbia, Canada, respectively [14].

The estimated incidence of tuberculosis was relatively higher than NTM associated diseases in hematological patients [2]. In a cohort of 2984 hematological patients, incidences of tuberculosis and NTM associated diseases were 1.78% and 1.2%, respectively [2]. Among the various subtypes of hematological malignancies, adult patients with acute myeloid leukemia (AML) had a significantly higher incidence of tuberculosis than other subtypes of hematological malignancies [1-3]. In areas with endemic MTB infections, acute lymphoblastic leukaemia was reported to be the most common malignancy in the pediatric oncology [19]. Ku et al. reported eight of 350 hematopoietic stem cell transplant recipients (HSCT) had pulmonary tuberculosis over a 6-year period [20]. The relative risk of having pulmonary tuberculosis after HSCT was 13.1-fold higher than in the general population. Incidences of tuberculosis and NTM associated diseases among various subtypes of hematological malignancies are shown in Figure 1 [2].

The incidence of NTM associated diseases in patients with hematological malignancies is not available in current literature. Among various species of NTM, *Mycobacterium avium-intracellulare* complex is the most commonly isolated NTM species (38%) in patients with hematological malignancies, followed by *M. abscessus* (21%), *M. fortuitum* (18%), and *M. kansasii* (18%) [2]. There is no difference of incidence and species of NTM associated infections in febrile neutropenia among patients with various subtypes of hematological malignancies [2].

Clinical Manifestation

Tuberculosis most commonly affects the lungs. It is transmitted from person to person via droplets from the throat and lungs of patients with active respiratory disease. In healthy people, infection with MTB often causes no symptoms, since patient's immune system acts to "wall off" the bacteria. Once the immune system breakdown, active tuberculosis occurred. Cough with purulent sputum or hemoptysis, chest pain, weakness, body weight loss, fever and night sweats are common symptoms of active pulmonary tuberculosis. Because patients with hematologic malignancy have impaired cellular immunity, they may present with atypical clinical symptoms and signs with MTB and NTM associated diseases [21-24].

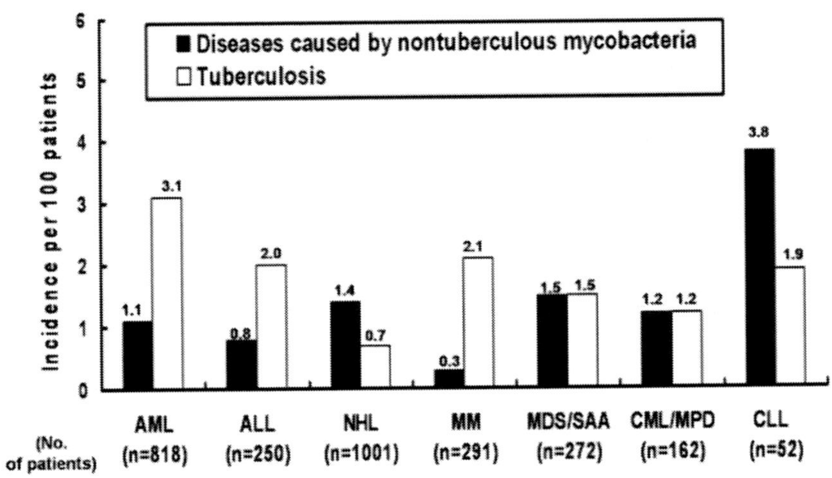

Figure 1. Incidence of diseases due to nontuberculous mycobacteria or *Mycobacterium tuberculosis* among patients with hematological malignancy at the National Taiwan University Hospital between 2001 and 2010. There were no differences in NTM infection among different hematological subtypes ($p = 0.445$). AML, acute myeloid leukemia; ALL, acute lymphoid leukemia; NHL, lymphoma; MDS, myelodysplastic syndrome; SAA, severe aplastic anemia; CML, chronic myeloid leukemia; MPD, myeloproliferative neoplasm; CLL, chronic lymphoid leukemia.

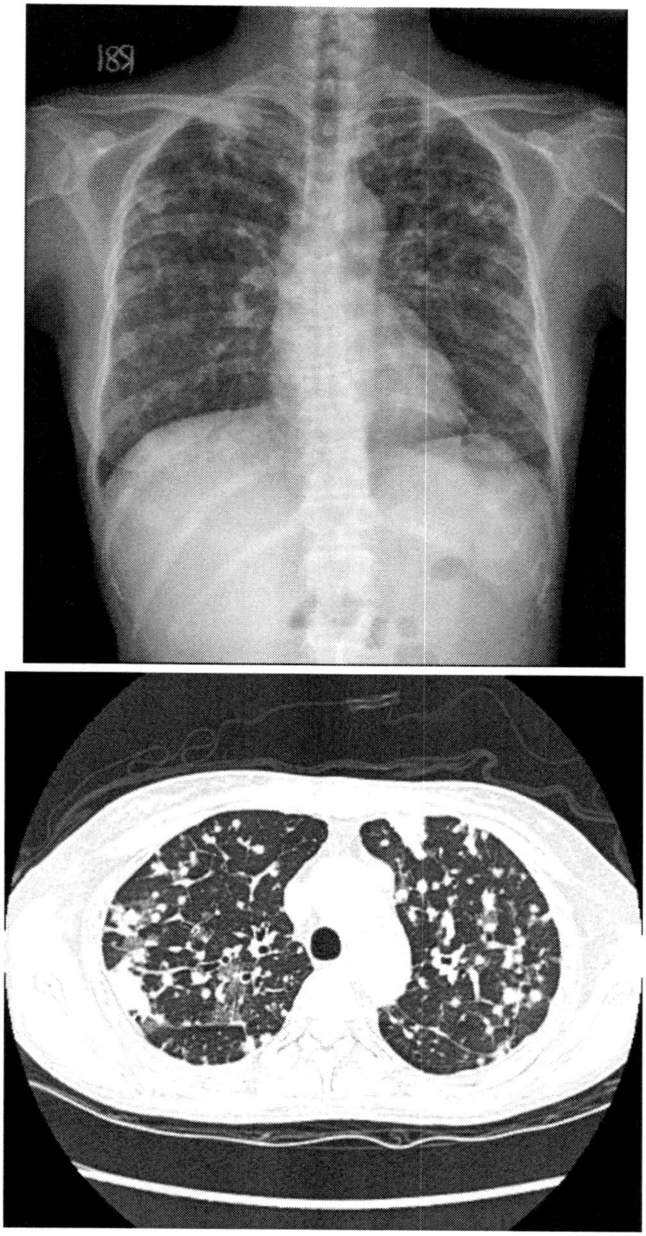

Figure 2. Pulmonary tuberculosis in a patient with AML and matched unrelated donor allogeneic transplantation (plain chest film and CT scan).

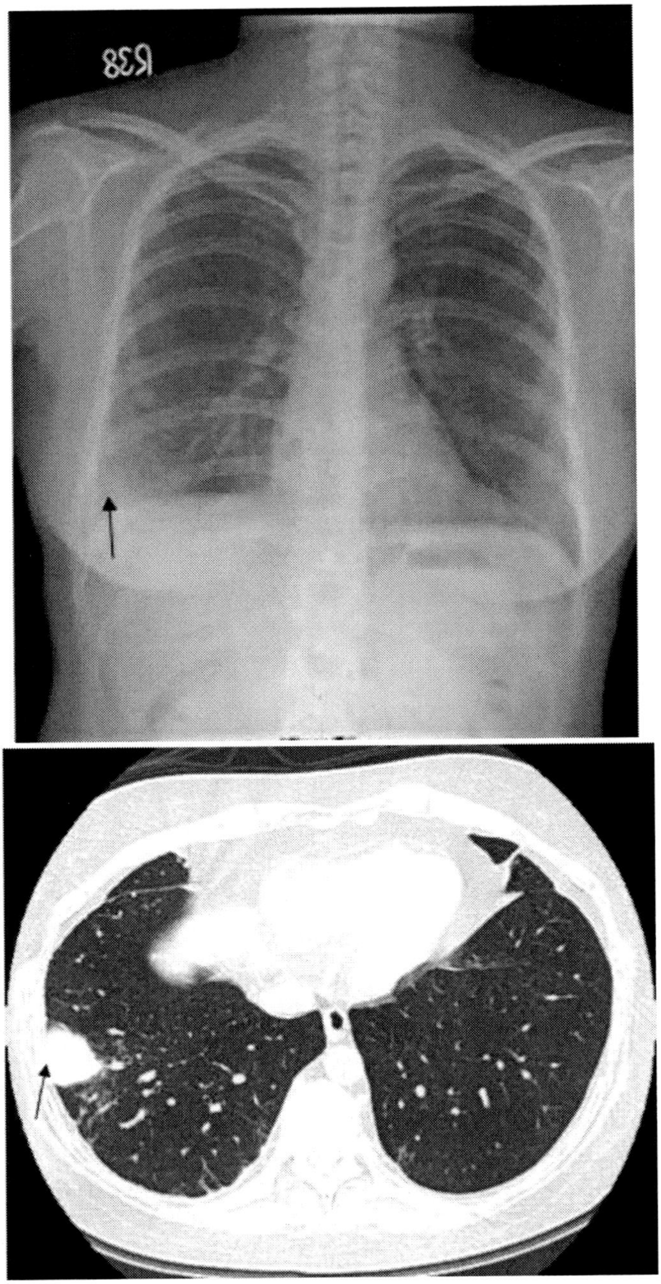

Figure 3. A 36-year-old woman with refractory AML. There is a right lower lobe nodule at plain chest film and CT scan. Biopsy showed both aspergillus and mycobacterium tuberculosis.

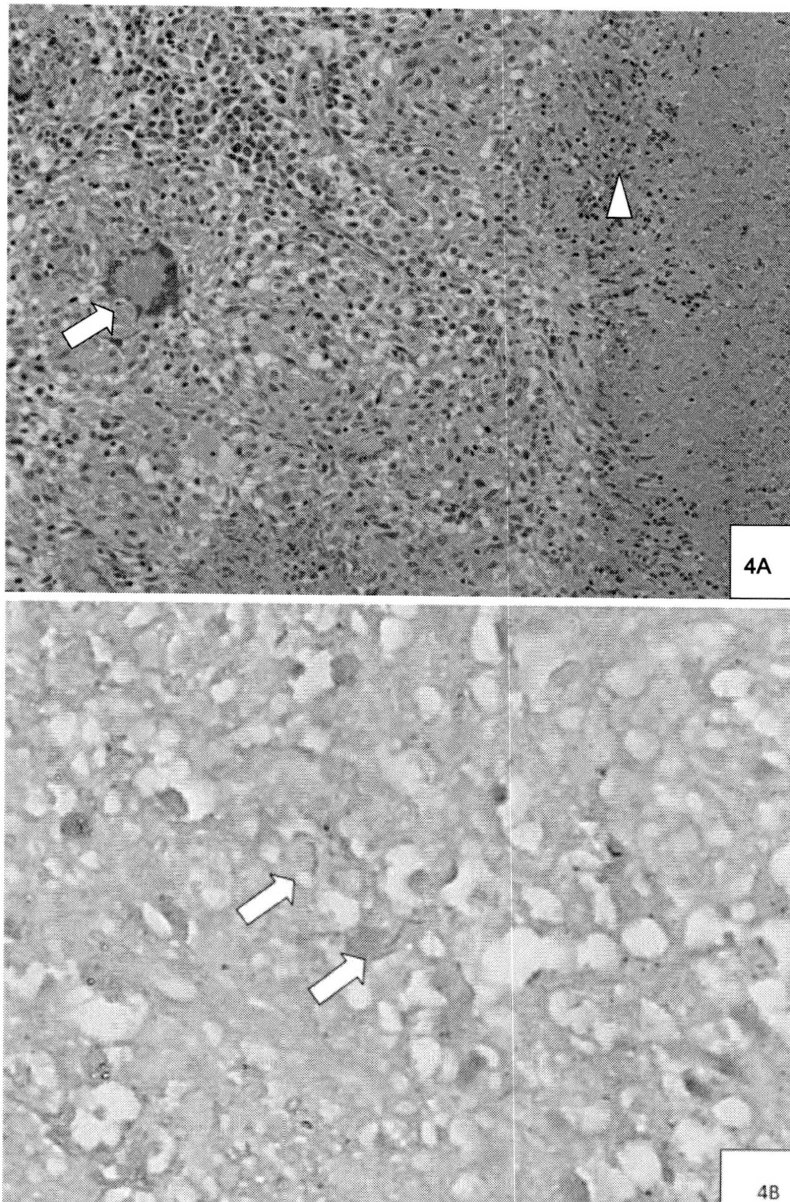

Figure 4. Pathological finding showed caseous necrosis and granuloma in lung tissue (H & E stain, 20X). 4A. Necrotizing granuloma in lung shows typical caseating necrosis (arrowhead) surrounded by epithelioid histiocytes and multinucleated giant cell (arrow). 4B. A few acid-fast bacilli (arrows) are demonstrated in area of caseating necrosis (Ziehl-Neelsen stain, original magnification x400).

Pulmonary Tuberculosis and NTM

Lung is the most commonly involved site of tuberculosis among cancer patients. The clinical symptoms and signs of tuberculosis in patients with hematological malignancies are heterogeneous and have varying severity. Most hematological patients have cough, sputum and fever. Tuberculosis could not be easily differentiated from NTM diseases or other opportunistic infections just by symptoms, signs and images. For example, a 47-year-old woman with underlying acute myeloid leukemia received matched- unrelated donor allogeneic transplantation. She had lung chronic graft versus host disease (GVHD) and was receiving tacrolimus. She had spiking fever up to 39°C productive cough more than three weeks while receiving broad spectrum antibiotics. Plain chest film and computed tomography (CT) are shown (Figure 2). Bilateral pulmonary infiltrations at chest plain film and CT scan showed multiple nodular lesions. Sputum acid-fast stain was positive for MTB and sputum culture finally yielded MTB. Her spiking fever gradually subsided one week after anti-MTB treatment Graft versus host disease (GVHD), idiopathic pneumonitis, and opportunistic infection such as cytomegalovirus, *Pneumocystis jiroveci*, fungi, and MTB or NTM are some of pulmonary complications in hematopoietic stem cell transplantation recipient. A detail history taking of tuberculosis exposure and examination of sputum for acid-fast bacilli and culture may improve the diagnostic accuracy [20, 25]. A 36-year-old woman with refractory AML developed spiking fever, pleuritic pain and non-productive cough after salvage chemotherapy. Her plain chest film and CT scan showed right lower lobe nodule (Figure 3). Pulmonary invasive fungal infection was considered first due to wedge shape nodule at chest CT scan. However, fever persisted while receiving broad-spectrum antibiotics and antifungal agents. Video-assisted wedge resection showed both fungal invasion and granulomatous inflammation with caseous necrosis and Langhans-type giant cells (Figure 4). This case demonstrated that tuberculosis could be co-infection with invasive fungal infection (such as aspergillosis) in the severe immunocompromised hematological patients.

Although reactivation of tuberculosis may happen in hematologic malignancy patients receiving chemotherapy by presentation of subacute or chronic clinical courses [3]. However, some patient may go through severe sepsis and a rapid fatal event [26]. The clinico-laboratory manifestations of hematological patients with tuberculosis are in Table 2. Most of hematological patients have pulmonary tuberculosis [3], and mediastinal lymphadenopathy (53%), pleural effusion (47%) and fibrocalcific lesions (43%) on chest imaging are the common presentations (Table 3) [3]. Since tuberculosis may mimic other diseases clinical and radiological presentations [27], sputum acid-fast stain and TB culture should be checked in any clinical suspicion of tuberculosis.

NTM are acid-fast bacilli commonly found in soil, water, and aerosols [28, 29]. These micro-organisms can inhabit body surfaces or secretions and have the ability to cause clinically insignificant colonization. NTM Pulmonary diseases should be only diagnosed when patient's clinical, radiological, and microbiological findings meet the American Thoracic Society (ATS) /Infectious Diseases Society of America (IDSA) criteria [30]. Briefly, the minimum evaluation of a patient suspected of NTM associated pulmonary disease should include the following: First, a chest radiograph or, in the absence of cavitation, chest high-resolution computed tomography (HRCT) scan; Second, three or more sputum specimens for acid-fast bacilli (AFB) analysis; and exclusion of other disorders, such as tuberculosis.

Patients with NTM associated pulmonary diseases usually have destructive pulmonary diseases, impaired host immunity such as in hematopoietic cell transplantation [31-34] and leukemia [35-37]. Most hematological patients with NTM associated disease are limited to pulmonary infection [2]. Symptoms and signs of NTM associated diseases are similar to tuberculosis, and cough, sputum, low grade fever and dyspnea are the most common clinical manifestation. Other opportunistic infections have the same clinical presentations and should be included into the differential diagnosis list. Characteristics of 34 patients with hematological malignancy and infections caused by NTM are shown in Table 4 [2].

Extrapulmonary Tuberculosis and NTM

Extrapulmonary tuberculosis is reported in 13%-58% of all tuberculosis [38-42]. Females have higher risk than males to acquire extra-pulmonary tuberculosis and have more tendencies for lymph node involvement [38-42]. It has been reported that extrapulmonary tuberculosis involves 28% of all tuberculosis in patients with hematological malignancies [3]. Pleural effusion is the most common manifestation of extrapulmonary tuberculosis, followed by lymphadenitis, bone and joints, urogenital, and central nervous system involvement. Extra-pulmonary tuberculosis is a diagnostic challenge for radiologist and particularly in high-risk population requires a high index of suspicion [43].

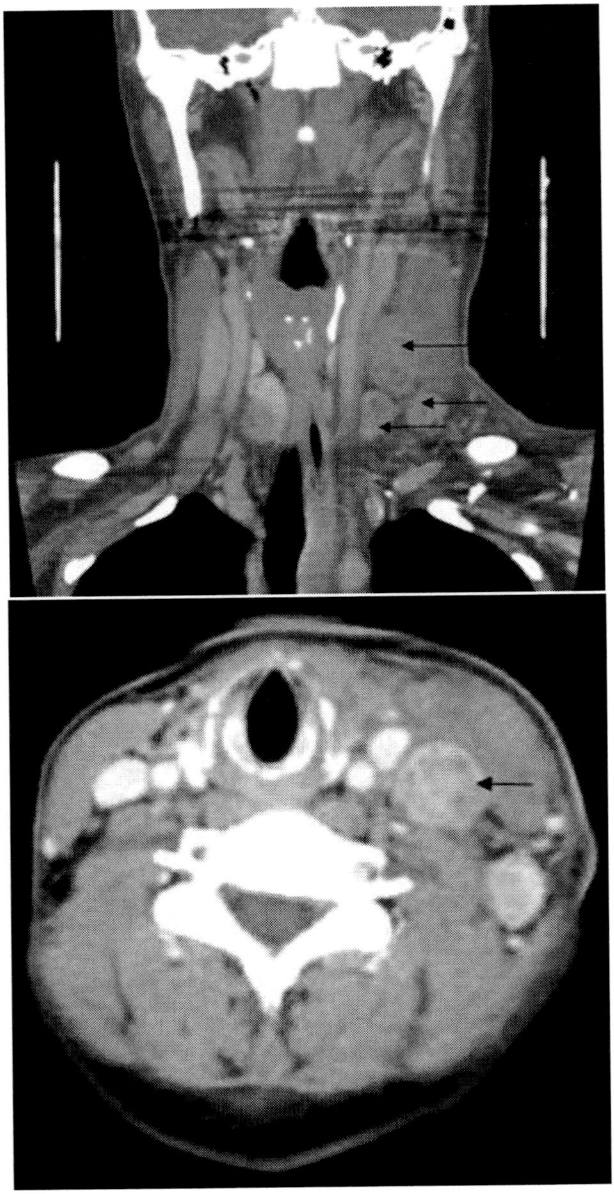

Figure 5. Extrapulmonary presentation of tuberculosis in a patient with acute myeloid leukemia (TB lymphadenitis) (Lymph node: arrow).

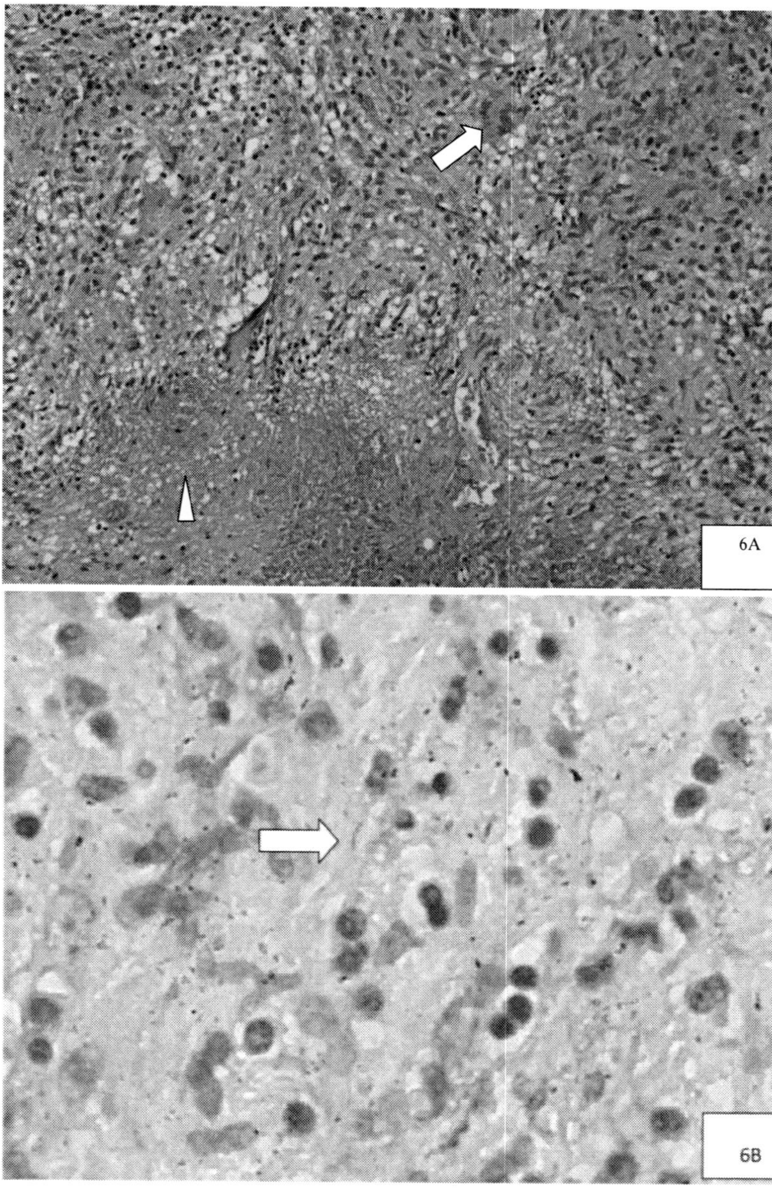

Figure 6. Pathological finding of caseous necrosis and granuloma formation in lymph node (H & E stain, 400X). 6A. Lymph node biopsy shows granulomatous inflammation characterized by clustered epithelioid histiocytes, multinucleated giant cells (arrow), and caseating necrotic debris (arrowhead). 6B. One acid-fast bacillus is identified by Ziehl-Neelsen stain (original magnification x400).

Table 2. Clinical and laboratory manifestations of 53 patients with hematological malignancy and *Mycobacterium tuberculosis* (MTB) infection

	Total (n = 53)	Neutropenia			Sites of tuberculosis		
		No (n = 27)	Yes (n = 26)	*P* value	Pulmonary TB only (n = 38)	Extra-pulmonary involvement[e] (n = 15)	*P* value
Elderly				.28			.24
Age more than 60 year	25	15	10		20	5	
Age less than 60 year	28	12	16		18	10	
Gender				.56			.34
Male	37	20	17		28	9	
Female	16	7	9		10	6	
Underlying Diabetes mellitus				.67			.66
Yes	6	4	2		5	1	
No	47	23	24		33	14	
Hematological Disease				.013			.76
Acute myeloid leukemia	29	10	19		20	9	
Non-Acute myeloid leukemia	24	17	7		18	6	
Diagnosis of tuberculosis and malignancy				.001			.33
Synchronous[a]	17	3	14		14	3	
Non-synchronous	36	24	12		24	12	
Allogeneic stem cell transplantation				.19			> .99
Yes	6	5	1		4	2	
No	47	25	22		34	13	
Defeverence within 72 hours[b]				.55			.030
Yes	17	9	8		15	2	
No	31	13	18		18	13	
Extra-pulmonary tuberculosis				> .99			
Yes	38	19	19				
No	15	8	7				

	Total (n = 53)	Neutropenia			Sites of tuberculosis		
		No (n = 27)	Yes (n = 26)	*P* value	Pulmonary TB only (n = 38)	Extra-pulmonary involvement[e] (n = 15)	*P* value
Laboratory data[c]							
Absolute neutrophil count (/uL) at fever	1970	3587	198	.019	2174	1100	.87
Absolute neutrophil count (/uL) at nadir	39	761	17	<. 001	39	39	.59
Albumin (g/dL)	3.60	3.48	3.70	.40	3.50	3.6	.80
Serum alanine aminotransferase (IU/L)	30	26	34	.67	34	27	.44
Alkaline phosphatase (IU/L)	174	207	141	.06	175	153	.52
Lactate dehydrogenase (IU/L)	509	574	440	.96	509	509	.58
C-reactive protein (mg/dL)	5.42	5.43	5.16	.60	5.59	4.73	.48
Treatment[d]				> .99			.048
Standard therapy	39	20	19		31	8	
Fluoroquinolone based therapy	9	4	5		4	5	
Outcome (30 days)				.61			.019
Death	3	1	2		0	3	
Alive	50	26	24		38	12	

Note: [a] Synchronous define as diagnosis of tuberculosis within 3 months of hematological malignancy.
[b] Five patients with pulmonary tuberculosis did not present with fever. [c] Median Value.
[d] Forty-eight patients received anti-tuberculosis treatment. [e] Five out of the 15 patients (33.3%) with extra-pulmonary tuberculosis (lymph node, 2; liver aspirates, 1; urine, 1; and blood, 1) also had documented pulmonary tuberculosis.

In MTB epidemic area, extra-pulmonary tuberculosis should be alerted as potential causes of febrile neutropenia among patients with hematological malignancies during chemotherapy. A 50-year-old woman with relapsing acute myeloid leukemia developed fever and several tender neck lymph nodes

4 weeks after re-induction chemotherapy. Plain chest film was normal. Magnetic resonance imaging of the neck is shown (Figure 5). Lymph node biopsy revealed caseating granulomatous inflammation with epitheliod cells and palisading multinucleated giant cells. Acid-fast stain revealed many acid-fast bacilli in the center of caseous necrosis (Figure 6). Lymph node culture confirmed MTB. Peripheral tuberculous lymphadenitis accounts for 10% of tuberculosis cases in the United States [44]. Female to male ratio is 1.4:1, with a peak age range of 30-40 years, and mostly in people who are born in MTB endemic areas [44]. Definitive diagnosis is by culture or nucleic amplification of MTB. Demonstration of acid fast bacilli and granulomatous inflammation may be helpful. Excisional biopsy has the highest sensitivity of 80%, but fine-needle aspiration is less invasive and especially in immunocompromised hosts and in resource-limited settings may be useful [44, 45].

Table 3. Radiological characteristics of 43 patients with pulmonary tuberculosis

Radiological findings	**Total (n = 43) (%)**	**Chest Plain film only (n = 14)**	**Chest CT scan (n = 29)**	***P* value**
Mediastinal and/or hilar lymphadenopathy	23 (53)	1	22	<. 001
Pleural effusion	20 (47)	5	15	.35
Fibrocalcified lesion	14 (43)	2	12	.095
Nodules	16 (37)	4	12	.51
Ground glass	6 (14)	0	6	.16
Pericardial effusion	6 (14)	0	6	.16
Interstitial pattern	2 (7)	1	1	> .99
Cavitation	2 (7)	0	2	> .99

Extra-pulmonary tuberculosis may also present as liver abscess. A 55-year-old man with refractory acute myeloid leukemia developed fever after salvage chemotherapy without definite infectious focus. An abscess was found at septic survey by abdominal CT scan (Figure 7). Echo guided biopsy and pathological report showed mixed acute and chronic inflammation with granulation tissue formation. MTB confirmed by abscess culture. Chronic disseminated candidiasis is a common complication of hematological malignancies, and usually involves liver, spleen, and kidney [46-48].

Hepatosplenic tuberculosis may mimic disseminated candidiasis in patients with acute leukemia [49].

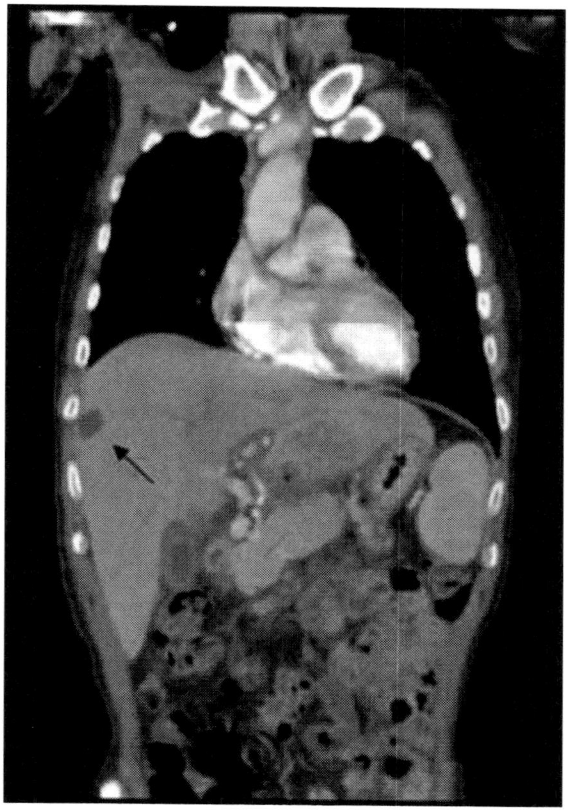

Figure 7. Extrapulmonary presentation of tuberculosis: Liver tuberculous abscess in a patient with acute myeloid leukemia.

A 45-year-old female presented with dyspnea and fever as initial manifestation of acute myeloid leukemia. Massive pericardial effusion was found in CT scan but there was no right atrium or right ventricle collapse sign (Figure 8). Pericardial effusion was drained by pigtail catheter, and pericardial fluid culture demonstrated tuberculosis four weeks after initiation of induction chemotherapy. The incidence of tuberculosis is increasing in non-industrialized countries [50, 51], and rarely reported in hematological patients [52]. Malignant pericardial effusion is occasionally found in patients with lymphoid malignancy, but it is rare in myeloid malignancy. Tuberculous pericarditis is a differential diagnosis of pericardial effusion in tuberculosis endemic region.

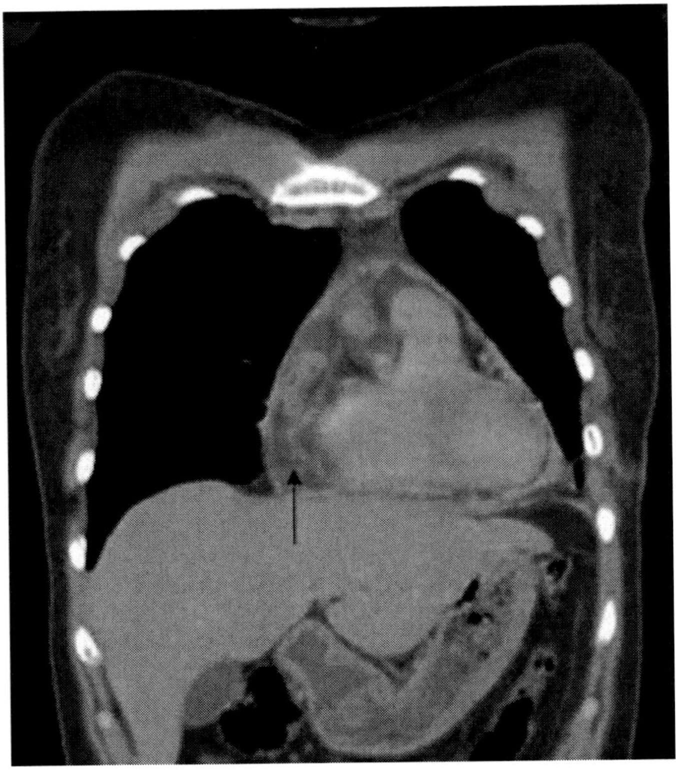

Figure 8. Extrapulmonary presentation of tuberculosis: Tuberculous pericardial effusion in a patient with acute myeloid leukemia.

A 53-year-old male with underlying chronic lymphocytic leukemia, had right knee swelling, tenderness and fever for several weeks. Bone scan demonstrated increased uptake in right knee (Figure 9). Culture of knee joint aspirate revealed *mycobacterium tuberculosis*. Diagnosis of musculoskeletal tuberculosis remains a challenge for clinicians and requires a high index of suspicion. Combination of indolent onset of symptoms and compatible radiographic findings strongly suggest the diagnosis. However, positive culture or histologic proof from the synovial fluid aspirate or synovial or bone biopsy must confirm TB. Prompt diagnosis and treatment of skeletal TB are important to prevent serious bone and joint destruction and severe neurologic sequelae in case of spinal involvement [53, 54].

One-fourth of tuberculosis among hematological patients has extra-pulmonary involvement [3]. Patients with extra-pulmonary TB disease usually have lower rates of defervescence within first 72 hour of empirical antimicrobial therapy (13% vs 45%, $p = 0.03$) compared to those with disease confined to the lungs [3]. Median duration of fever in patients with extra-pulmonary tuberculosis is longer than those with disease confined to the lungs (15 days vs 9 days, $p = 0.025$).

A 30-year-old male with chronic phase of chronic myeloid leukemia had fever, cough, and multiple mediastinal lymph nodes. CT scan of the chest was significant with multiple mediastinal lymphadenopathy mimic tumor (Figure 10). Sputum and lymph node culture was positive for *mycobacterium kansasii*. Disseminated NTM-infection may *mimic* tumor on CT scan [55].

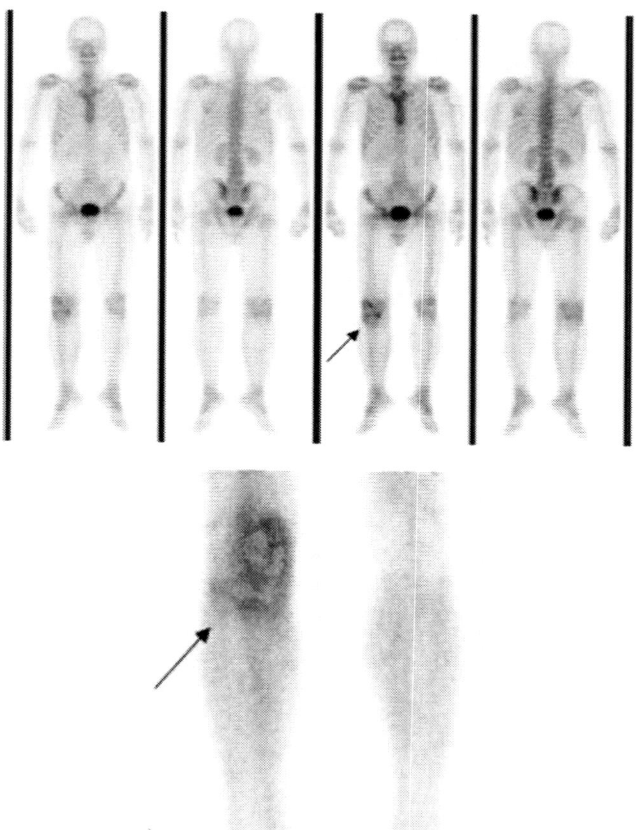

Figure 9. Right knee arthritis noted by bone scan, culture yield mycobacterium tuberculosis.

Table 4. Characteristics of 34 patients with hematological malignancy and infections caused by nontuberculous mycobacteria

Characteristics	Total (n = 34)	Pulmonary only (n = 26)	Disseminated (n = 8)	*P* value
Age median (range) year	57 (18-86)	57 (18-56)	43 (28-79)	0.417
Gender				0.066
Male	26	20	4	
Female	8	6	4	
Hematological malignancy remission status				0.645
Yes	8	7	1	
No	26	19	7	
Stem cell transplantation				0.645
Yes	8	7	1	
No	26	19	7	
Neutropenia				0.007
Yes	5	1	4	
No	29	25	4	
Underlying disease				
Diabetes mellitus	2	1	1	0.421
Chronic liver disease	2	2	0	> 0.999
Chronic kidney disease	4	3	1	> 0.999
Steroid use	21	17	4	0.699
Autoimmune disease	2	2	0	> 0.999
Old pulmonary tuberculosis	4	4	0	0.551
Initially adequate antibiotic treatment				0.403
Yes	25	18	7	
No	9	8	1	
30-day outcome				0.570
Survivors	29	23	6	
non-Survivors	5	3	2	

A 38-year-old female presented with fever, jaundice and pancytopenia. T/NK lymphoma with hemophagocytosis was confirmed by pathology and flow cytometry. She had persistent fever under broad spectrum antibiotics, intravenous immunoglobulin. Patient gradually developed altered level of mental status and leptomeningeal enhancement was found in magnet resonance imaging (MRI) (Figure 11). Sputum, bone marrow and cerebrospinal fluid culture was positive for *M. kansasii.* Diversity of severity and clinical manifestations is problematic in diagnosis of NTM associated disease in patients with hematological malignancies.

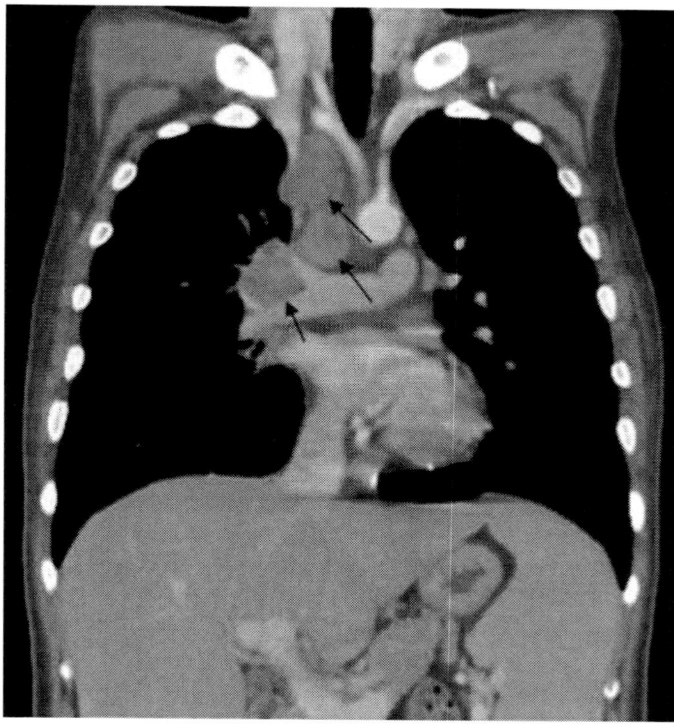

Figure 10. A 30-year-old man with underlying chronic phase of chronic myeloid leukemia had fever, cough, and multiple mediastinal lymph nodes. Culture yields *mycobacterium kansasii.*

One fourth of patients with hematological malignancies and NTM have disseminated disease with multiple organ involvement such as bone marrow, liver, spleen, lymph nodes, central nervous system and gastrointestinal tract. At the time of diagnosis, neutropenia is more frequent in patients with disseminated NTM than patients with pulmonary NTM disease [2]. Patients with NTM associated diseases have higher absolute neutrophil counts at diagnosis and a higher 30-day mortality rate (15% vs. 2%) than TB patients. Chronic kidney disease and severe neutropenia (absolute count < 500/μl) at the time of diagnosis were independent prognostic factors of NTM associated diseases in patients with hematological malignancy.

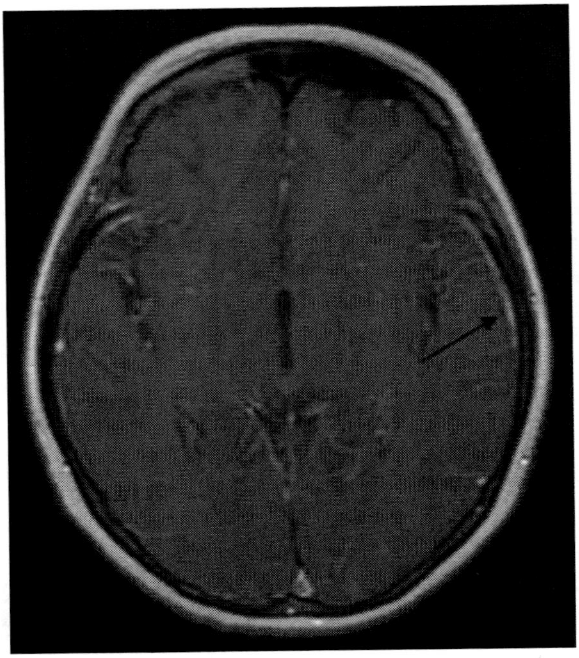

Figure 11. A 38-year-old woman with T/NK lymphoma, hemophagocytosis had disseminated mycobacterium kansasii infection. MRI (T1) showed leptomengingeal enhancement.

Neutropenia

Since neutrophils have short life span, are easily activated, and cannot be cryopreserved, the *in vitro* study has variable results [56]. Furthermore, the accuracy of studies examining neutrophil-mycobacteria interaction, rarely characterized in patients with isolated or depleted granulocytes. It has been suggested that neutrophil have several functions in tuberculosis, including early clearance of infection, human neutrophil peptides mediated mycobacteria killing, phagocytosis enhanced by antibodies, influence on acquired immune response, and neutrophil-mediated inflammation and tissue damage in active disease [56]. Neutrophils are the most commonly infected phagocytes in the airway infection by tuberculosis [57]. A prospective study was done on active TB patients, latent TB patients and/or positive *M. tuberculosis* antigen-specific tuberculin skin test to improve TB diagnosis, and extent of the disease. This study demonstrated that a 393 transcript signature, a neutrophil-driven interferon-inducible gene profile, in patients with active TB correlates with radiological extent of disease [58]. Neutrophils are less well studied compare to other components of host response to MTB infection and probably in part because of inherent difficulties in working with these cells in basic studies, most of the available data is controversial [56].

Increased utilization of anti-neoplastic agents in treatment of hematological malignancies is associated with an increase of endemic opportunistic infections such as tuberculosis. Neutropenia and impaired humoral and cellular immunity are frequent complications in patients with hematological malignancies. A prospective study of 130 patients with acute leukemia demonstrated that patients with AML rather than ALL had a higher rate of tuberculosis [1]. Similar results support the observation that adult AML patients might have a relatively higher rate of tuberculosis than other types of hematologic malignancies [3]. Since neutrophil counts were unknown in previous studies [1, 28], we discovered that compared to non-AML patients, tuberculosis in AML patients is often associated with significant febrile neutropenia (66% vs. 29%, $p = 0.013$) [3]. Risk of acquiring tuberculosis may partly correlate with patient's absolute neutrophil count, but this association may not apply to all different types of hematological malignancies.

Recent studies on human neutrophil peptides has highlighted their bactericidal action against MTB and suggested that neutrophils may play a more important defensive role in tuberculosis [59]. Neutrophils may mediate innate immunity against mycobacterium. A study of people who have been exposed to a patient with active TB demonstrated that neutrophils make a significant contribution in host defense against *M. tuberculosis.* In this study, higher neutrophil count was associated with more resistance to early infection with MTB, and risk of tuberculosis was inversely and independently associated with peripheral blood neutrophil counts in people who had contact with pulmonary tuberculosis patients [60]. This study was consistent with other studies and supporting the important role of neutrophils in defense against MTB infection. MTB and NTM associated disease can be an important differential diagnosis for patients with hematological malignancies who present with febrile neutropenia.

The timing of reactivation or development of tuberculosis in patients with hematological malignancies is not clear. Since 43% of patients with hematological malignancies had fibrocalcified lesions on the chest CT, we conclude that most patients might have had old TB infection before febrile neutropenia [3]. Impaired immunity by underlying hematological malignancies and/or chemotherapy induced immunosuppression may lead to reactivation of tuberculosis in patients with hematological malignancies. It is not clear when patients may develop active tuberculosis, and needs further prospective investigation [3].

Neutrophils play an important role in controlling tuberculosis in human blood [61]. Absolute neutrophil count is significantly lower in patients with MTB than those patients with NTM associated diseases [2]. Clinical manifestations of tuberculosis and gram negative bacilli infection in hematological patients with febrile neutropenia was compared as bellow. Twenty-six patients with tuberculosis at febrile neutropenia were compared with the 52 hematological disease status matched patients with *K. pneumoniae* infections at febrile neutropenia (Table 5). Clinically, patients with tuberculosis showed a significant lower rate of hypotension at the onset of fever (0% vs. 19%, $p = 0.026$) and after a longer duration of fever (10.5 days vs. 3.0 days, $p < 0.001$). From the laboratory results, patients with tuberculosis showed higher white blood cell counts (median, 198 vs. 0, $p < 0.001$) and absolute neutrophil counts (median, 17 vs. 0, $p = 0.046$) at the leucopenia nadir stage than patients with *K. pneumoniae* infections. Although the 30-day mortality of patients with MTB disease is lower than that of patients with *K. pneumoniae* infections (30-day mortality rates, 8% vs. 17%), the difference is not statistically significant ($p = 0.319$).

Diagnosis

Chest X radiographs are commonly use as screening for pulmonary tuberculosis, while sputum acid-fast stains and cultures are the gold standard of tuberculosis confirmation. In a retrospective study, sputum acid-fast stains and cultures were performed in all 53 patients with hematological malignancy (median 3 sets, ranged 1-14). Of the 43 patients culture proved pulmonary tuberculosis, sputum smear for acid-fast was positive only in nine patients (21%). Sputum smear was negative in the remaining 34 patients [3]. In another retrospective study, *acid-fast stain* was positive in seven out of 34 patients with *NTM associated diseases* (21%) [2]. Fifteen out of 53 patients with hematological malignancy (28%) had extra-pulmonary disease, with positive cultures from lymph nodes (n = 4), liver aspirates (n = 3), synovial fluid (n = 2), ascites (n = 2), urine (n = 2), abdominal wall abscess (n = 1), and blood (n = 1). In the same study, five out of 15 patients (33.3%) with extra-pulmonary tuberculosis (2 patients in lymph nodes, one patient in liver aspirate, one patient in urine and one patient in blood) also had concomitant pulmonary tuberculosis. Caesous necrosis and granuloma may be found both in MTB and NTM associated disease, and the definite diagnosis depends on culture results.

Many studies have assessed the value of in-house nucleic-acid amplification tests for diagnosis of tuberculosis, but absence of reproducibility makes it difficult to assess these tests [8]. However, several commercial nucleic-acid amplification tests for tuberculosis are available. These tests generally have high specificity, and sensitivity is high in smear-positive sputum but is less than that of culture. Nucleic acid amplification tests have little value other than confirming that the acid-fast bacilli are MTB *[62]. Nucleic-acid amplification tests in smear-negative sputum or extrapulmonary disease have limited value owing to their moderate sensitivity, and cultures still need to be done [8].*

Interferon-gamma-release assays (IGRAs) are alternatives to the tuberculin skin test (TST). Recent meta-analysis demonstrated that IGRAs especially Quantiferon Gold tests have high specificity which is not affected by tuberculin skin test [63, 64]. However, patients with hematological malignancies frequently have impaired cellular immunity, and role of interferon gamma release assays in these patients still is not clear. In a study, ten patients with hematological malignancies (AML, 5; lymphoma, 4; multiple myeloma, 1; myelodysplastic syndrome, 1) and febrile neutropenia, blood interferon gamma release assay was done. Three patients who had AML and positive assay had culture-confirmed pulmonary tuberculosis. The other 7 patients with negative assay were all culture-negative for MTB or TB ruled out. However, the data of interferon-gamma-release assays is very limited in patients with hematological malignancies, and still need large scale investigation.

A retrospective study of patients with hematological malignancies and newly detected unexplained pulmonary lesion on chest CT demonstrated that 3.8% of tuberculosis diagnosed by CT guided biopsy was undiagnosed in patients with hematological malignancies and pulmonary lesions [65]. Pulmonary infiltration is a frequent presentation of tuberculosis in cancer patients, but chest x ray findings was not suggestive of TB in 20% of patients [66]. Although nonspecific pneumonia is one of the radiographic findings of pulmonary tuberculosis, it is not helpful for diagnosis. In our retrospective study, most patients with hematological malignancies and pulmonary tuberculosis had mediastinal lymphadenopathy, pleural effusions, and fibrocalcified lesions [3]. Reactivation of tuberculosis owing to immunocompromised status secondary to hematological malignancies and /or chemotherapy associated neutropenia is common and should be highly suspected. It has been suggested that lymphadenopathy is the most characteristic radiological feature of primary tuberculosis. Hilar and mediastinal lymph nodes with a central hypodense area in enhanced CT of the chest support diagnosis [67]. However, only few patients have the typical presentation of mediastinal lymph node with central hypodense lesion. This characteristic image finding is not sensitive enough to predict pulmonary tuberculosis [3]. CT scan of the chest reveals mediastinal lymphadenopathy in half of patients with pulmonary tuberculosis, and can be a better predictor of culture positive tuberculosis. Computer tomography is significantly better at discovering mediastinal lymphadenopathy ($p < 0.001$) than plain chest radiography [2, 3]. Hence, CT of the chest may be a more valuable tool for diagnosing pulmonary tuberculosis in patients with hematological malignancies and respiratory symptoms and signs after chemotherapy.

Treatment

Isoniazid, rifampin, ethambutol, pyrazinamide, and streptomycin are five antimicrobial agents that are currently recommended as first-line anti-tuberculosis therapy [68]. Extensive studies of these drugs have shown the favorable therapeutic ratios [69, 70]. Cycloserine, clofazimine, ethinamide, and para-aminosalicylic acid are the second-line medications, and either have been shown to be less effective and more toxic or have not been studied more extensively than the first-line agents. There are some reports concerning drug resistance of MTB in patients with hematological malignancies. In a retrospective study 81% of patients received standard anti-tuberculosis treatment (isoniazide, rifampin, ethambutol, and pyrazinamide) and fluoroquinolone based anti-tuberculosis therapy was given to19% of patients. Drug resistance was noticed in 17.0% of patients with MTB, and one isolate (1.9%) was resistant to both isoniazid and rifampin (multi-drug resistant MTB) [3]. The drug resistance percentages were as stated for isoniazid ($n = 5$, 9.4%), streptomycin ($n = 4$, 7.5%), rifampin ($n = 1$, 1.9%) and ethambutol ($n = 1$, 1.9%) [3].

The polymorphonuclear leukocytes (PMN) have important role in the early stages of tuberculosis. In an *in vitro* study, the effects of four anti TB medications (rifampicin, isoniazid, pyrazinamide and ethambutol) examined separately and together on the functions of human PMN [71]. Flow cytometric techniques were used to compare PMN phagocytosis and oxidative burst with and without incubation in different concentrations of the drugs. Flow cytometry did not show any influence of these drugs on PMN phagocytosis. Only the highest concentrations of isoniazid and of the combined drugs could attenuate oxidative burst comparing to lower concentrations. This study demonstrated that PMN function deterioration observed in MTB disease is probably due to MTB and irrelevant to the anti-TB treatment.

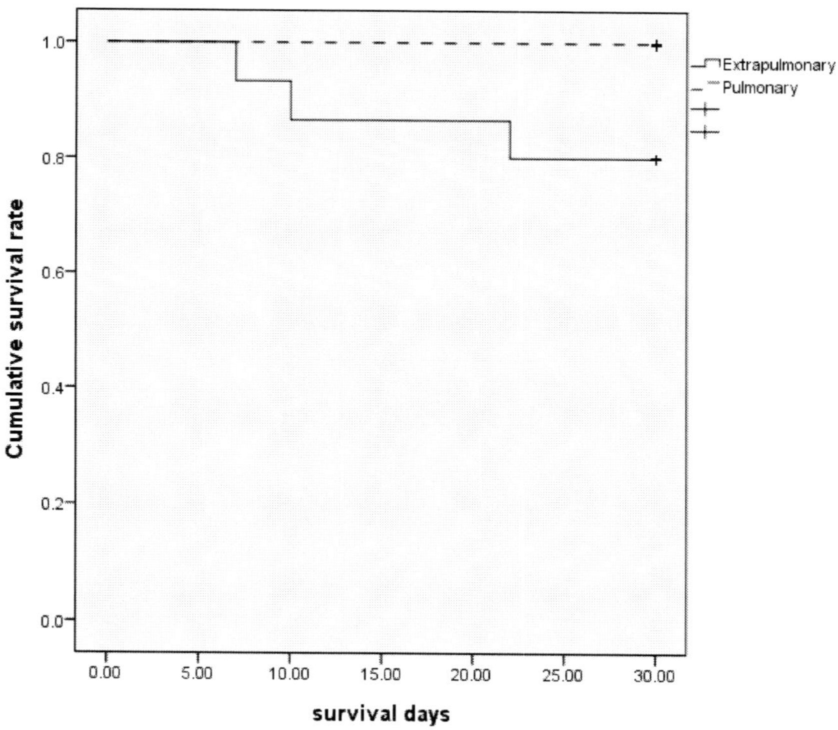

Figure 12. 30-day mortality between pulmonary and extra-pulmonary tuberculosis (p = 0.004).

Recognition of the current role of NTM isolates remains the key step in NTM infections management [35, 72]. After diagnosis, treatment must be guided by the isolated species, specific syndromes, clinical experience and results of in-vitro susceptibility tests. Surgical intervention may be considered for some species (*Mycobacterium ulcerans, Mycobacterium scrofulaceum*) and localized infections. Treatment of uncommon species is not yet well defined and recent studies on resistance mechanisms have described their importance [35, 72]. Extra-pulmonary NTM such as cervicofacial lymphadenitis frequently treated with surgical resection [73, 74]. Patients with hematological malignancy usually have neutropenia and increased bleeding tendency. Surgical resection of NTM associated diseases is limited in clinical practices.

Table 5. Case-control comparison of clinical laboratory characteristics in hematological malignancies with tuberculosis and Klebsiella pneumoniae infection during febrile neutropenia

	Patients with tuberculosis infection (n = 26)	**Patients with Klebsiella pneumoniae infection (n = 52)**	***P* value**
Elderly			0.187
Age more than 60 year	10	12	
Age less than 60 year	16	40	
Gender			0.335
Male	17	27	
Female	9	25	
Underlying Diabetes mellitus			0.597
Yes	2	2	
No	24	50	
Hematological Disease			1.000
Acute myeloid leukemia	19	38	
Non-Acute myeloid leukemia	7	14	
Disease status			0.093
Remission	3	16	
Active hematological disease	23	36	
Allogeneic stem cell transplantation			1.000
Yes	1	2	
No	25	50	
Hypotension at fever			0.026
Yes	0	10	
No	26	42	
Duration of fever* (Day)	10.5	3.0	< 0.001
Duration of neutropenia* (Day)	12	13.0	0.764
Laboratory data*			
White blood cell count at fever onset* (/ul)	1185	240	0.004
White blood cell count at nadir* (/ul)	315	70	0.102
Absolute neutrophil count at fever onset* (/ul)	198	0	< 0.001

	Patients with tuberculosis infection (n = 26)	Patients with Klebsiella pneumoniae infection (n = 52)	*P* value
Absolute neutrophil count at nadir* (/ul)	17	0	0.046
Albumin* (g/dl)	3.70	3.80	0.401
Serum GPT* (IU)	34	36	0.395
Alkaline phosphatase* (IU)	141	157	0.471
BUN* (mg/dl)	12.65	15.75	0.115
Creatinine* (mg/dl)	0.9	0.8	0.941
LDH* (IU)	440	364	0.830
CRP*	5.16	6.48	0.229
Outcome (30 days) 0.319			
Death	2	9	
Alive	24	43	

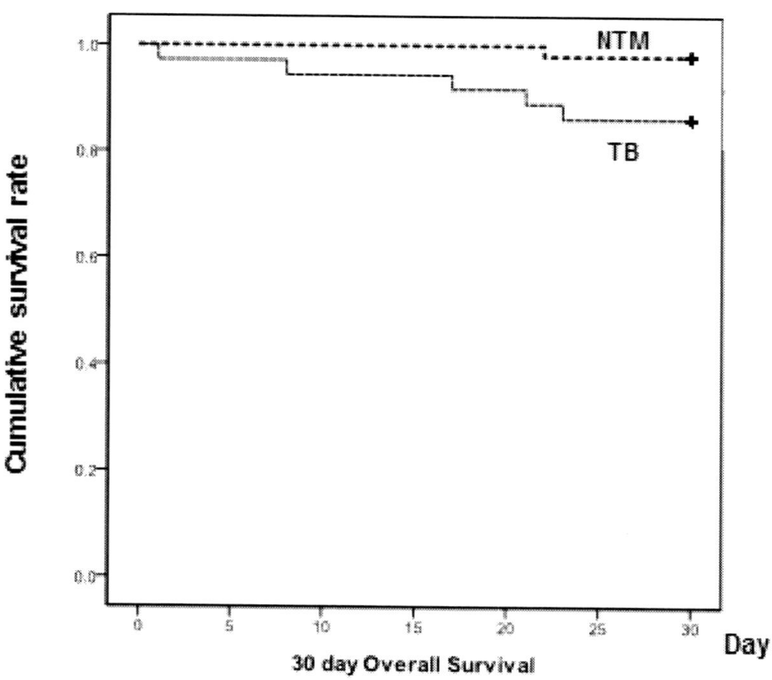

Figure 13. Comparison of 30-day overall survival between patients with hematological malignancy and tuberculosis (TB) and patients with infections caused by nontuberculous mycobacteria (NTM) (Kaplan-Meier analysis, log rank test, $p = 0.025$).

Table 6. Comparisons of clinical characteristics of patients with hematological malignancy and tuberculosis with patients with infections caused by nontuberculous mycobacteria (NTM)

Characteristic	No. (%) of patients NTM infection (n = 34)	Tuberculosis (n = 50)	*P* value
Age: ≥ 60 years	14 (41)	24 (48)	0.656
< 60 years	20 (59)	26 (52)	
Gender: Male	26 (76)	35 (70)	0.305
Female	8 (24)	15 (30)	
Remission: Yes	8 (24)	6 (12)	0.233
No	26 (76)	44 (88)	
Allogeneic stem cell transplant: Yes	8 (24)	4 (8)	0.060
No	26 (76)	46 (92)	
Diabetes mellitus: Yes	2 (6)	6 (12)	0.464
No	32 (94)	44 (88)	
Chronic liver disease: Yes	2 (6)	2 (4)	> 0.999
No	32 (94)	48 (96)	
Chronic Kidney disease: Yes	4 (12)	5 (10)	> 0.999
No	30 (88)	45 (90)	
Steroid use: Yes	21 (62)	26 (52)	0.502
No	13 (38)	24 (48)	
Radiological finding*			
Cavitation: Yes	3 (9)	2 (4)	0.390
No	31 (91)	48 (96)	
Fibrosis: Yes	7 (21)	15 (30)	0.450
No	27 (79)	35 (70)	
Nodules: Yes	13 (38)	15 (30)	0.484
No	21 (62)	35 (70)	
Pulmonary opacity: Yes	21 (61)	6 (12)	< 0.001
No	13 (38)	37 (74)	
Laboratory finding at diagnosis			
White blood cell count (median, uL)	7205	4630	0.233
Absolute neutrophil count (median, uL)	4114	1970	0.003
Albumin (g/dl)	3.5	3.7	0.581
Lactate dehydrogenase (IU/L)	489	500	0.105
C-reactive protein (mg/dL)	6.08	5.09	0.075

Treatment for NTM associated diseases in patients with hematological malignancies is also under investigation. In our retrospective study, 10 out of

13 patients (77%) with MAC infection received adequate initial antibiotic treatment. Three patients received clarithromycin, ethambutol, and rifabutin, four patients received isoniazid, rifampin, ethambutol, and pyrazinamide, and fluoroquinolone and/or imipenem were given to three patients [2]. Four out of 6 patients with *M. kansasii* infection were received adequate initial antibiotic treatment. Two patients received clarithromycin, ethambutol, and rifabutin, one patient received isoniazid, rifampin, ethambutol, and pyrazinamide, and quinolone and imipenem were given to one patient. Ten out of 14 patients (71%) with rapidly growing mycobacteria (*M. abscessus, M. fortuitum,* and *M. chelonae*) received adequate initial antibiotic treatment. Four patients received clarithromycin and ciprofloxacin, three patients received imipenem and/or amikacin, and quinolone-based antibiotics were given to three patients. In total, 25 out of 34 patients (74%) were received adequate initial antibiotic treatment. However, adequate initial antibiotic treatment was not associated with a decline in 30-day mortality ($p = 0.391$).

Outcome

Overall mortality of tuberculosis in patients with hematological malignancy is 2-11% [1-3]. In a prospective study of 130 consecutive patients with acute leukemia, 9 patients had active TB and only one patient died with disseminated tuberculosis during post induction neutropenia [1]. All other eight patients were successfully managed using current anti-tuberculous therapy. Patients with hematological malignancy and extra-pulmonary tuberculosis disease usually have a higher 30-day in-hospital mortality compared to those with disease confined to the lungs (20% vs. 0%, $p = 0.004$) [3]. The result is shown in Figure 11.

NTM associated disease have 20% mortality in patients with hematological malignancy [2]. In a retrospective study, we compared 30-day mortality of patients with NTM with MTB associated diseases. Five out of 34 (15%) NTM patients died within 30 days after clinical diagnosis of NTM infection, but only one out of (2%) 50 tuberculosis patients died within 30 days. Kaplan-Meier analysis revealed that patients with hematological malignancy and NTM diseases have significantly worse outcome than patients with tuberculosis (log rank test, $p = 0.025$, Figure 12) [2].

Conclusion

Patients with hematological malignancy and neutropenia have higher risk of developing MTB and NTM associated diseases. Epidemiology of MTB in patients with hematological malignancy and neutropenia is still under investigation. Clinical and radiological manifestations can especially be atypical in patients with extra-pulmonary involvement. Acid-fast stain and culture are the standard method for detecting MTB and NTM. First-line anti-tuberculosis agents such as isoniazid, rifampin, ethambutol and pyrazinamide can most of the time effectively controls the disease. NTM associated diseases should be treated according to the isolated mycobacterial species, and surgical resection may be needed in some patients with extra-pulmonary infection.

References

[1] Mishra P., Kumar R., Mahapatra M., Sharma S., Dixit A., Chaterjee T., Choudhry D. R., Saxena R., Choudhry V. P. Tuberculosis in acute leukemia: A clinico-hematological profile. *Hematology.* 2006; 11: 335-40.

[2] Chen C. Y., Sheng W. H., Lai C. C., Liao C. H., Huang Y. T., Tsay W., Huang S. Y., Tang J. L., Tien H. F., Hsueh P. R. Mycobacterial infections in adult patients with hematological malignancy. *Eur J Clin Microbiol Infect Dis.* 2012; 31:1059-66.

[3] Chen C. Y., Sheng W. H., Cheng A., Tsay W., Huang S. Y., Tang J. L., Chen Y. C., Wang J. Y., Tien H. F., Chang S. C. Clinical characteristics and outcomes of Mycobacterium tuberculosis disease in adult patients with hematological malignancies. *BMC Infect Dis.* 2011; 11:324.

[4] Gupta A., Singh M., Singh H., Kumar L., Sharma A., Bakhshi S., Raina V., Thulkar S: Infections in acute myeloid leukemia: An Analysis of 382 febrile episodes. *Med Oncol* 2010, 27:1037-45.

[5] Shamsi T. S., Irfan M., Ansari S. H., Farzana T., Khalid M. Z., Panjwani V. K., Baig M. I., Shakoor N. Allogeneic peripheral blood stem cell transplantation in patients with haematological malignancies. *J Coll Physicians Surg Pak* 2004, 14:522-526.

[6] Centers for Disease Control and Prevention (CDC). Trends in tuberculosis- United States, 2011. *MMWR Morb Mortal Wkly Rep.* 2012; 61:181-5.

[7] Hsueh P. R., Liu Y. C., So J., Liu C. Y., Yang P. C., Luh K. T. Mycobacterium tuberculosis in Taiwan. *J Infect.* 2006; 52:77-85.

[8] World Health Organization. http://www.who.int/mediacentre/factsheets/fs104/en/.

[9] Kamboj M., Sepkowitz K. A. The risk of tuberculosis in patients with cancer. *Clin Infect Dis.* 2006; 42: 1592-5.

[10] Kato S., Ito K., Takatorige T., Ohkado A., Tanaka K., Ishikawa N. Medical service systems for tuberculosis in low-incidence countries. *Kekkaku.* 2012; 87: 577-84.

[11] Oxlade O., Murray M., Tuberculosis and poverty: Why are the poor at greater risk in India? *PLoS One.* 2012; 7: e47533.

[12] World Health Organization. http://www.who.int/tb/publications/global_report/gtbr12_annex2.pdf.

[13] Moore J. E., Kruijshaar M. E., Ormerod L. P., Drobniewski F., Abubakar I. Increasing reports of non-tuberculous mycobacteria in England, Wales and Northern Ireland, 1995-2006. *BMC Public Health.* 2010; 10: 612.

[14] Hernández-Garduño E., Rodrigues M., Elwood R. K. The incidence of pulmonary non-tuberculous mycobacteria in British Columbia, Canada. *Int J Tuberc Lung Dis.* 2009; 13: 1086-93.

[15] Khan K., Wang J., Marras T. K. Nontuberculous mycobacterial sensitization in the United States: national trends over three decades. *Am J Respir Crit Care Med* 2007; 176: 306-313.

[16] Marras T. K., Chedore P., Ying A. M., Jamieson F. Isolation prevalence of pulmonary non-tuberculous mycobacteria in Ontario, 1997- 2003. *Thorax* 2007; 62: 661-666.

[17] Simons S., van Ingen J., Hsueh P. R., van Hung N., Dekhuijzen P. N., Boeree M. J. et al., Nontuberculous mycobacteria in respiratory tract infections, eastern Asia. *Emerg Infect Dis* 2011; 17: 343-349.

[18] Lai C. C., Tan C. K., Chou C. H., Hsu H. L., Liao C. H., Huang Y. T. et al., Increasing incidence of nontuberculous mycobacteria, Taiwan, 2000-2008. *Emerg Infect Dis* 2010; 16:294-296.

[19] Stefan D. C., Kruis A. L., Schaaf H. S., Wessels G. Tuberculosis in oncology patients. *Ann Trop Paediatr.* 2008; 28: 111-116.

[20] Ku S. C., Tang J. L., Hsueh P. R., Luh K. T., Yu C. J., Yang P. C. Pulmonary tuberculosis in allogeneic hematopoietic stem cell transplantation. *Bone Marrow Transplant* 2001; 27: 1293-1297.

[21] Kaplan M. H., Armstrong D., Rosen P: Tuberculosis complicating neoplastic disease. A review of 201 cases. *Cancer* 1974, 33:850-858.

[22] Al-Anazi K. A., Al-Jasser A. M., Evans D. A. Infections caused by mycobacterium tuberculosis in patients with hematological disorders and in recipients of hematopoietic stem cell transplant, a twelve year retrospective study. *Ann Clin Microbiol Antimicrob.* 2007; 6: 16.

[23] Maartens G., Wilkinson R. J., Tuberculosis. *Lancet* 2007, 370: 2030-2043.

[24] Kobashi Y., Mouri K., Yagi S., Obase Y., Miyashita N., Okimoto N., Matsushima T., Oka M. Clinical features of immunocompromised and nonimmunocompromised patients with pulmonary tuberculosis. *J Infect Chemother* 2007, 13:405-410.

[25] Cordonnier C., Martino R., Trabasso P., Held T. K., Akan H., Ward M. S., Fabian K., Ullmann A. J., Wulffraat N., Ljungman P., Alessandrino E. P., Pretnar J., Gmür J., Varela R., Vitek A., Sica S., Rovira M. European Blood and Marrow Transplant Group Infectious Diseases Working Party. Mycobacterial infection: a difficult and late diagnosis in stem cell transplant recipients. *Clin Infect Dis* 2004; 38: 1229-1236.

[26] Ker C. C., Hung C. C., Sheng W. H., Chang S. C., Luh K. T. Fatal mycobacteremia caused by Mycobacterium tuberculosis in a patient with acute leukemia. *Leukemia.* 1999; 13: 646-7.

[27] Burrill J., Williams C. J., Bain G., Conder G., Hine A. L., Misra R. R. Tuberculosis: a radiologic review. *Radiographics.* 2007; 27: 1255-73.

[28] Wagner D., Young L. S. Nontuberculous mycobacterial infections: A clinical review. *Infection* 2004; 32: 257-270.

[29] Jarzembowski J. A., Young M. B. Nontuberculous mycobacterial infections. *Arch Pathol Lab Med* 2008; 132: 1333-1341.

[30] Griffith D. E., Aksamit T., Brown-Elliott B. A., Catanzaro A., Daley C., Gordin F. et al. An official ATS/IDSA statement: Diagnosis, treatment, and prevention of nontuberculous mycobacterial diseases. *Am J Respir Crit Care Med* 2007; 175: 367-416.

[31] Doucette K., Fishman J. A. Nontuberculous mycobacterial infection in hematopoietic stem cell and solid organ transplant recipients. *Clin Infect Dis* 2004; 38: 1428-1439.

[32] Au W. Y., Cheng V. C., Ho P. L., Yuen K. Y., Hung I., Ma S. Y. et al., Nontuberculous mycobacterial infections in Chinese hematopoietic stem cell transplantation recipients. *Bone Marrow Transplant* 2003; 32: 709-14.

[33] Almyroudis N. G., Fabian J., Hahn T., Segal B. H., Wetzler M., McCarthy P. L. Jr. Late infectious complications after cord blood stem

cell transplantation. *Eur J Clin Microbiol Infect Dis* 2009; 28: 1405-1408.

[34] Weinstock D. M., Feinstein M. B., Sepkowitz K. A., Jakubowski A. High rates of infection and colonization by nontuberculous mycobacteria after allogeneic hematopoietic stem cell transplantation. *Bone Marrow Transplant* 2003; 31: 1015-1021.

[35] Levendoglu-Tugal O., Munoz J., Brudnicki A., Fevzi Ozkaynak M., Sandoval C., Jayabose S. Infections due to nontuberculous mycobacteria in children with leukemia. *Clin Infect Dis* 1998; 27:1227-1230.

[36] Suryanarayan K., Campbell J., Eskenazi A. E. Nontuberculous mycobacterial infections in pediatric acute leukemia. *J Pediatr Hematol Oncol* 2002; 24:558-560.

[37] Damsker B., Bottone E. J., Deligdisch L. *Mycobacterium xenopi*: Infection in an immunocompromised host. *Hum Pathol* 1982; 13: 866-870.

[38] Noertjojo K., Tam C. M., Chan S. L., Chan-Yeung M. M. Extra-pulmonary and pulmonary tuberculosis in Hong Kong. *Int J Tuberc Lung Dis.* 2002; 6: 879-86.

[39] Al-Otaibi F., El Hazmi M. M. Extra-pulmonary tuberculosis in Saudi Arabia. *Indian J Pathol Microbiol.* 2010; 53: 227-31.

[40] García-Rodríguez J. F., Álvarez-Díaz H., Lorenzo-García M. V., Mariño-Callejo A., Fernández-Rial Á., Sesma-Sánchez P. Extrapulmonary tuberculosis *Enferm Infecc Microbiol Clin.* 2011; 29: 502-9.

[41] Ozvaran M. K., Baran R., Tor M., Dilek I., Demiryontar D., Arinç S., Toker N., Chousein E. U., Soğukpinar O. Extrapulmonary tuberculosis in non-human immunodeficiency virus-infected adults in an endemic region. *Ann Thorac Med.* 2007; 2: 118-21.

[42] Lin J. N., Lai C. H., Chen Y. H., Lee S. S., Tsai S. S., Huang C. K., Chung H. C., Liang S. H., Lin H. H. Risk factors for extra-pulmonary tuberculosis compared to pulmonary tuberculosis. *Int J Tuberc Lung Dis.* 2009; 13: 620-5.

[43] Maclean K. A., Becker A. K., Chang S. D., Harris A. C. Extrapulmonary Tuberculosis: Imaging Features beyond the Chest. *Can Assoc Radiol J.* 2012 Dec 22.

[44] Fontanilla J. M., Barnes A., von Reyn C. F. Current diagnosis and management of peripheral tuberculous lymphadenitis. *Clin Infect Dis.* 2011; 53: 555-62.

[45] Artenstein A. W., Kim J. H., Williams W. J., Chung R. C. Isolated peripheral tuberculous lymphadenitis in adults: Current clinical and diagnostic issues. *Clin Infect Dis.* 1995; 20: 876-82.

[46] Masood A., Sallah S. Chronic disseminated candidiasis in patients with acute leukemia: Emphasis on diagnostic definition and treatment. *Leuk Res.* 2005; 29: 493-501.

[47] Rammaert B., Desjardins A., Lortholary O. New insights into hepatosplenic candidiasis, a manifestation of chronic disseminated candidosis. *Mycoses.* 2012; 55: e74-84.

[48] Chen C. Y., Chen Y. C., Tang J. L., Yao M., Huang S. Y., Tsai W., Chen Y. C., Shen M. C., Wang C. H., Tien H. F. Hepatosplenic fungal infection in patients with acute leukemia in Taiwan: Incidence, treatment, and prognosis. *Ann Hematol.* 2003; 82: 93-7.

[49] Lee D. G., Choi J. H., Kim Y. J., Lee S., Min C. K., Kim D. W., Lee J. W., Min W. S., Shin W. S., Kim C. C. Hepatosplenic tuberculosis mimicking disseminated candidiasis in patients with acute leukemia. *Int J Hematol.* 2001; 73: 119-21.

[50] Mayosi B. M., Burgess L. J., Doubell A. F. Tuberculous pericarditis. *Circulation.* 2005; 112: 3608-16.

[51] Fowler N. O. Tuberculous pericarditis. *JAMA.* 1991; 266: 99-103.

[52] Russo R. L., Dulley F. L., Suganuma L., França I. L., Yasuda M. A., Costa S. F. Tuberculosis in hematopoietic stem cell transplant patients: Case report and review of the literature. *Int J Infect Dis.* 2010; 14 Suppl 3: e187-91.

[53] Yao D. C., Sartoris D. J. Musculoskeletal tuberculosis. *Radiol Clin North Am.* 1995; 33: 679-89.

[54] Grosskopf I., Ben David A., Charach G., Hochman I., Pitlik S. Bone and joint tuberculosis-a 10-year review. *Isr J Med Sci.* 1994; 30: 278-83.

[55] Lin K. H., Wang J. H., Peng N. J. Disseminated nontuberculous mycobacterial infection mimic metastases on PET/CT scan. *Clin Nucl Med.* 2008; 33: 276-277.

[56] Lowe D. M., Redford P. S., Wilkinson R. J., O'Garra A., Martineau A. R. Neutrophils in tuberculosis: Friend or foe? *Trends Immunol.* 2012; 33: 14-25.

[57] Eum S. Y., Kong J. H., Hong M. S., Lee Y. J., Kim J. H., Hwang S. H., Cho S. N., Via L. E., Barry C. E. 3rd. Neutrophils are the predominant infected phagocytic cells in the airways of patients with active pulmonary TB. *Chest.* 2010; 137: 122-8.

[58] Berry M. P., Graham C. M., McNab F. W., Xu Z., Bloch S. A., Oni T., Wilkinson K. A., Banchereau R., Skinner J., Wilkinson R. J., Quinn C., Blankenship D., Dhawan R., Cush J. J., Mejias A., Ramilo O., Kon O. M., Pascual V., Banchereau J., Chaussabel D., O'Garra A. An interferon-inducible neutrophil-driven blood transcriptional signature in human tuberculosis. *Nature.* 2010; 466: 973-7.

[59] Fu L. M., The potential of human neutrophil peptides in tuberculosis therapy. *Int J Tuberc Lung Dis* 2003, 7:1027-1032.

[60] Martineau A. R., Newton S. M., Wilkinson K. A., Kampmann B., Hall B. M., Nawroly N., Packe G. E., Davidson R. N., Griffiths C. J., Wilkinson R. J. Neutrophil-mediated innate immune resistance to mycobacteria. *J Clin Invest* 2007; 117: 1988-1994.

[61] Martineau A. R., Newton S. M., Wilkinson K. A., Kampmann B., Hall B. M., Nawroly N., Packe G. E., Davidson R. N., Griffiths C. J., Wilkinson R. J. Neutrophil-mediated innate immune resistance to mycobacteria. *J Clin Invest.* 2007; 117: 1988-94.

[62] Piersimoni C., Scarparo C. Relevance of commercial amplification methods for direct detection of *Mycobacterium tuberculosis* complex in clinical samples. *J Clin Microbiol,* 2003; 41: 5355–5365.

[63] Pai M., Zwerling A., Menzies D. Systematic review: T-cell-based assays for the diagnosis of latent tuberculosis infection: An update. *Ann Intern Med.* 2008; 149: 177-84.

[64] Lalvani A., Millington K. A. T cell-based diagnosis of childhood tuberculosis infection. *Curr Opin Infect Dis.* 2007; 20: 264-71.

[65] Gupta S., Sultenfuss M., Romaguera J. E., Ensor J., Krishnamurthy S., Wallace M. J., Ahrar K., Madoff D. C., Murthy R., Hicks M. E. CT-guided percutaneous lung biopsies in patients with haematologic malignancies and undiagnosed pulmonary lesions. *Hematol Oncol.* 2010; 28: 75-81.

[66] Libshitz H. I., Pannu H. K., Elting L. S., Cooksley C. D. Tuberculosis in cancer patients: An update. *J Thorac Imaging* 1997; 12: 41-46.

[67] Andreu J., Caceres J., Pallisa E., Martinez-Rodriguez M. Radiological manifestations of pulmonary tuberculosis. *Eur J Radiol* 2004; 51: 139-149.

[68] Small P. M., Fujiwara P. I. Management of tuberculosis in the United States. *N Engl J Med.* 2001; 345: 189-200.

[69] Fox W., Ellard G. A., Mitchison D. A. Studies on the treatment of tuberculosis undertaken by the British Medical Research Council

tuberculosis units, 1946-1986, with relevant subsequent publications. *Int J Tuberc Lung Dis.* 1999 Oct; 3(10 Suppl 2): S231-79.

[70] *Tuberculosis chemotherapy including directly observed therapy.* In: Iseman MD. A clinician's guide to tuberculosis. Philadelphia: Lippincott Willims & Wilkins, 2000:271-321. 69.

[71] Kielland L. G., Vage R. A., Eide G. E., Sørnes S., Naess A. Anti-tuberculosis drugs and human polymorphonuclear leukocyte functions. *Chemotherapy.* 2011; 57(4): 339-44.

[72] Esteban J., García-Pedrazuela M., Muñoz-Egea M. C., Alcaide F. Current treatment of nontuberculous mycobacteriosis: An update. *Expert Opin Pharmacother.* 2012; 13: 967-86.

[73] Mandell D. L., Wald E. R., Michaels M. G., Dohar J. E. Management of nontuberculous mycobacterial cervical lymphadenitis. *Arch Otolaryngol Head Neck Surg.* 2003; 129: 341-4.

[74] Lindeboom J. A. Surgical treatment for nontuberculous mycobacterial (NTM) cervicofacial lymphadenitis in children. *J Oral Maxillofac Surg.* 2012; 70:345-8.

In: Neutropenia
Editors: M. Akhtari et al.
ISBN: 978-1-63482-105-6

Chapter 6

Syndrome of Cocaine-Levamisole-Induced Asculopathy and Eutropenia

***Samuel H. Poon*[1] *and Anthony M. Reginato*[2]**
[1]Division of Rheumatology, Roger William Medical Center,
Providence Veterans Administration Medical Center,
Rhode Island Hospital and Warren Alpert School of Medicine
at Brown University, Providence, RI, US
[2]Providence Veterans Administration Medical Center,
Rhode Island Hospital and Warren Alpert School of Medicine
at Brown University, Providence, RI, US

Introduction

Levamisole, an adulterant in street cocaine, is increasingly recognized amongst health care providers since 2009 when it became known that 70% of the seized cocaine within the United States borders contained this agent [1]. Levamisole was introduced as an anthelminthic for human use in 1966, and was further investigated for use in conditions ranging from pediatric nephrotic syndrome, colon cancer, to rheumatoid arthritis (RA) [2-4]. Adverse reactions attributed to levamisole use had been known since early 1970s, with severe agranulocytosis being the most concerning, which led to its withdrawal from the United States market in 2000 [5]. In 2006, reports of severe neutropenia associated with cocaine use began surfacing. In January 2009, the New Mexico Department of Health (NMDOH) detected levamisole using gas chromatography/mass spectrometry in a postmortem blood specimen from a patient who was deceased from *Serratia marcesans* sepsis related to neutropenia [1, 6]. By November 2009, a combined effort between epidemiologists at Seattle and King County Department of Public Health and the NMDOH identified 21 cases of cocaine associated agranulocytosis, from which 4 of 5 patients tested returned with positive levamisole [1]. Since that time, a novel rheumatic syndrome of levamisole-cocaine associated neutropenia and cutaneous vasculitis with positive anti-neutrophil cytoplasmic antibodies (ANCA) has been described. In this chapter, we will explore the pharmacologic profiles of levamisole and cocaine, review the clinical spectrum of this emerging autoimmune syndrome and discuss the therapeutic approach for management of its complications.

Levamisole as Therapy

A Lesson in History

Levamisole is the *levo* isomer of tetramisole, which was discovered in 1966 as an anthelminthic [7]. In invertebrates, levamisole (L-1[-1]-2,3,5,6-Tetrahydro-6-phenylimidazo[2,1b]-thiazole hydrochloride) acts as a nicotinic acetylcholine (ACh) agonist, thereby interfering with the muscle membrane of nematodes [8]. It continues to be a useful agent for the treatment of nematode infections in veterinary medicine, and is still prescribed in countries where parasitic infections are endemic [9]. Human use for this indication in the United States and Canada, however, had been discontinued since 2000 and 2003, respectively. Presently, levamisole is considered as a steroid-sparing agent and viable therapeutic option in children with steroid responsive nephrotic syndrome (SRNS) with frequent relapses outside of North America [10, 11].

During the late 1970s, more widespread use of levamisole was employed in the treatment of rheumatoid arthritis patients [12, 13]. It was thought to be an effective treatment for this disease until the observations of acute neutropenia and skin rashes were apparent. In a study of 60 patients with rheumatoid arthritis treated with levamisole, six developed severe neutropenia with polymorphonuclear counts less than 1.0×10^9 cells/L [12]. Use of levamisole for treatment of RA fell out of favor due to a lack of efficacy. In a double blind levamisole-placebo control study of 30 RA patients, one third of patients had recurrence after initial response and only 36% of patients treated with levamisole reached clinical remission. A significant number of patients (64%) experienced significant adverse events including secondary leukopenia or skin rash [14].

Another report in 1978 found that *in vitro* neutrophil chemotaxis from cells isolated from RA patients treated with this drug was enhanced above the baseline normal values, casting a question if levamisole had an immunostimulatory effect as opposed to an immunosuppressive one [Authors: this is a review not original article - corrected] [15]. Finally, levamisole was also used briefly as an adjuvant therapy for the treatment of colorectal cancer in the 1990s, until subsequent evidence demonstrated that adding levamisole to 5-fluorouracil (5-FU) failed to confer additional benefit [16].

Levamisole Immunology

Levamisole is an immunomodulator, which denotes an ability to either augment or suppress an immune response [17]. Similar to the 1978 study, subsequent studies solidified its profile as an immunostimulatory drug. Levamisole had been shown to inhibit T suppressor cell function, and to enhance IL-1 production, increase phagocytic activity of peritoneal macrophages, NK cell function, T cell and delayed type hypersensitivity response, and promote granulocyte maturation [17, 18]. Although levamisole may also act as a co-chemotherapeutic agent, these properties provide the rationale for its use as immunotherapy in colorectal cancer, and continue to be studied as a chemical adjuvant to boost hepatitis B and DNA-based cancer vaccine responses [18-20].

Despite the fact that levamisole had been shown primarily to be an immunostimulating agent, the mechanistic rationale for its use in SRNS and perhaps RA in the past may lie in the finding that it modulates the immune system by preferentially enhancing T helper type 1 (Th1) responses, and down-regulating type 2 (Th2) responses, that are felt to be the primary driver in the pathogenesis of SRNS [21].

Levamisole as an Adulterant in Cocaine

It continues to be unclear why levamisole had been added into street cocaine. Illicit drug manufacturers may "cut" levamisole into cocaine solely as a bulking agent. However, it has been postulated that levamisole affect CNS pathways via multiple mechanisms [5]. Mood elevation was a reported side effect when it was used in metastatic colon cancer treatment [22]. *In vitro* studies demonstrated that levamisole is a very weak partial agonist on human neuronal nicotinic ACh receptors [23]. Rather, levamisole exerts its CNS effects in the human nicotinic ACh system via non-competitive allosteric modulation on an alternate binding site [23]. It remains a leading hypothesis that levamisole had been intentionally added to cocaine for its mood altering effects, perhaps via neuronal nicotinic ACh receptors, to enhance cocaine euphoria [23, 24]. A lack of nicotinic symptoms from patients taking levamisole may be explained by the *in vitro* findings that levamisole acts via an alternative binding site for acetylcholinergic compounds modulating the effects of agonists/antagonists as opposed to direct agonistic activity [23].

In effect, levamisole changes the binding potential and ultimate biologic effects of known CNS nicotinic agonists such as nicotine, acetylcholine, or antagonists like cocaine [25]. Other theories include the selective inhibition of monoamine oxidase type A (MAO) and decreased norepinephrine reuptake resulting in the accumulation of a breakdown metabolite with amphetamine like effects, and increased endogenous opioid concentrations as seen in rat studies [24].

Levamisole Induced Agranulocytosis

Soon after its introduction as an immunoregulatory drug for the treatment of RA, cases of levamisole induced leukopenia and neutropenia were noted by observant clinicians. In a prospective placebo-controlled study, levamisole treatment led to persistent neutropenia in 35% of patients, and 6 out of 60 RA patients (10%) developed severe neutropenia (PMN less than $1x10^9$ cells/L) [12]. Fifteen patients (35% total) in the cohort were also found to have reduced neutrophil counts by greater than 30% for more than three months. The duration of exposure to levamisole was between one to 23 months in this study. Hematologic side effect of levamisole was reversible and recurred after repeated exposure. Bone marrow aspirates ranged from normal granulopoiesis to maturation arrest [12].

Interestingly, it has been demonstrated that there is an association between agranulocytosis, levamisole and MHC class I epitope HLA-B27 in RA patients, and in as high as 33-50% of cases of levamisole- associated neutropenia [26, 27]. In a recent study of 20 patients with levamisole agranulocytosis, three of five patients tested were positive for HLA-B27, whereas local population has a HLA-B27 prevalence of 8.5% [27].

The discovery that levamisole possibly causes agranulocytosis via an immune mechanism as opposed to direct bone marrow toxicity was evaluated in the early 1980s. Thompson et al. described ten patients between 48-70 years of age who became severely neutropenic after exposure to levamisole for either RA or breast cancer treatment [28]. Sera derived from these patients were shown to be granulocytoxic. This study determined that the IgM subclass of immunoglobulin was responsible for levamisole-induced granulocytopenia in three patients [28]. This finding had since been validated in a subsequent analysis of patients exposed to levamisole-tainted cocaine. In a study of patients with unexplained granulocytopenia, 70% of them were positive for recent or ongoing cocaine use. Three out of five cocaine associated patients (60%) were positive for anti-neutrophil antibodies and HLA-B27, although the immunoglobulin subtypes were IgM or IgG [27]. Bone marrow biopsy was normocellular marrow in 6/13 patients, but 9/13 patients had granulocyte hypoplasia, and megakaryocytes were increased in 10/13 patients [27]. It should be noted that presence of ANCA is not diagnostic for ANCA associated vasculitis (AAV) and one should consider levamisole-contaminated cocaine use.

Levamisole Induced Vasculitis

It has been reported that cutaneous vasculitis with complement consumption was present in a seropositive RA patient who was treated with levamisole. Leukocytoclastic vasculitis was present on skin biopsy, with IgM and complement deposition which disappeared after levamisole stopped [29]. As treatment with levamisole for pediatric SRNS continued in the 1990s, sporadic cases of levamisole associated cutaneous vasculitis were identified further. The lesions were characterized by a sudden onset of purpuric macules, which can expand to form plaques to hemorrhagic bullae. Cheeks and characteristically, external pinna and nose were frequently involved (Figure 1) [30-34].

Some patients experienced fever and arthralgia. Serologic testing showed positive ANCA in predominately perinuclear pattern, although anti-nuclear antibodies, and lupus anti-coagulant antibodies were positive in some patients. Cutaneous vasculitis resolved after withdrawal of the levamisole in these cases.

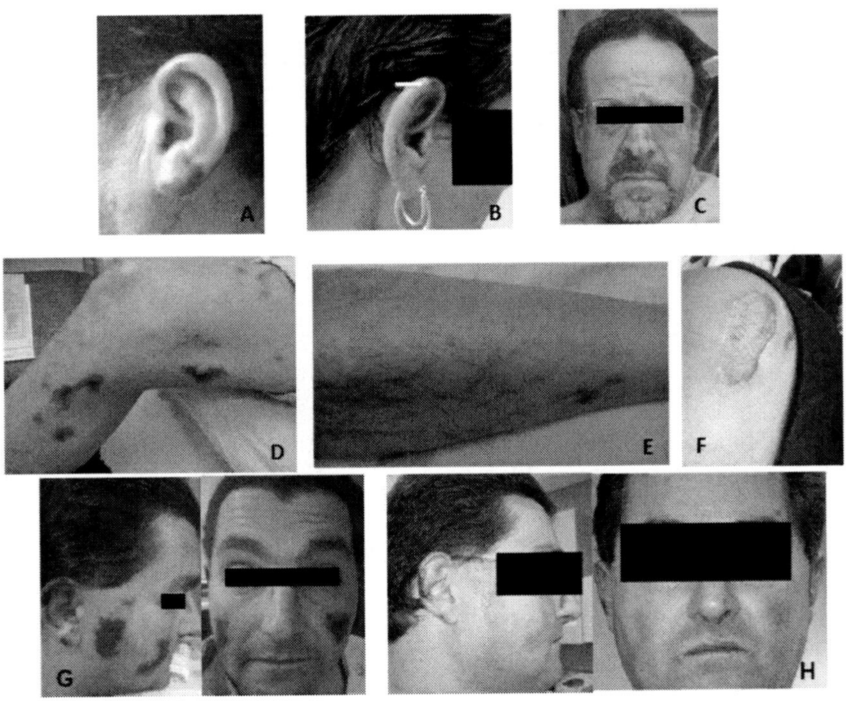

Figure 1. Cutaneous manifestations of levamisole-cocaine induced vasculitis. **(A, B)** Purpuric macules on the ears. **(C)** Purpuric macules on nasal dorsum. **(D, E)** Multiple stelate and purpuric plaques with early necrosis on the left lower leg. **(F)** Necrotic lesions in the knee. **(G)** Multiple purpuric lesions on cheeks (face) and pinna. **(H)** Healed lesions after treatment with prednisone.

Rheumatic Manifestations of Cocaine

Cocaine had been reported to cause multiple rheumatologic syndromes. These can range from Raynaud's phenomenon, chronic skin ulcers, cutaneous vasculopathy and vasculitis, urticarial vasculitis, necrotizing granulomatous vasculitis, to digital and limb necrosis [35]. Systemic vasculitic syndromes ranging from eosinophilic granulomatosis with polyangiitis/Churg-Strauss syndrome (EPA) to granulomatosis with polyangiitis/Wegener's granulomatosis (GPA) to cerebral vasculitis had been attributed to cocaine exposure [36-38]. Cocaine abuse is thought to lead to tissue ischemia due to its vasospastic and prothrombotic properties. Increasingly, pseudovasculitis with extensive inflammatory infiltration to frank vasculitis had been observed in cases where dermal vessels, oral mucosa, or brain parenchyma were analyzed histologically [36-38, 39, 40].

Perhaps the most well described rheumatic syndrome which is directly linked to chronic cocaine use is the syndrome of cocaine-induced midline destructive lesions (CIMDL) [41, 42]. CIMDL patients have nasal and palatal perforations leading to impressive midline sinonasal destruction. They present with chronic nasal obstruction, epistaxis, and severe facial pain. As repetitive trauma from chronic cocaine use can lead to sinus destruction, some patients may complain of dysphagia and nasal reflux due to progressive necrotic lesions [42]. This syndrome completely mimics GPA patients with "limited" presentations, outside of the clinical difference that patients with CIMDL do not have constitutional symptoms such as fever, malaise, weight loss, myalgias, or arthralgias [42]. Like patients with limited presentations of GPA, pulmonary, renal, and other systemic findings are absent. ANCA serologies are often positive in CIMDL patients, which were predominately in a perinuclear pattern. ELISA testing shows reactivity to PR3 in 48% of CIMDL patients. However, reactivity to anti-human elastase (HNE) is more specific in cocaine users (84% positive). Histopathologic studies of sinus biopsies seldom show granulomatous lesions, or true vasculitis findings in CIMDL, a further distinguishing feature which would be expected in GPA patients [43].

ANCA Associated Neutropenia and Drug Induced ANCA Vasculitis

Owing to the fact that both cocaine and levamisole had been shown to provoke reactivity to ANCA serologies and both had been associated with vasculitic lesions, two questions therefore arise. First, whether ANCA directly causes agranulocytosis. Second, whether levamisole-cocaine induced vasculitis represents a drug induced ANCA associated vasculitis (AAV) similar to propylthiouracil (PTU) induced AAV.

ANCA Associated Neutropenia

ANCA measures the presence of antibodies against cytoplasmic granules in ethanol fixed neutrophils. Myeloperoxidase (MPO) and proteinase 3 (PR3) are two specific cytoplasmic antigens with strong associations with GPA, EPA, and microscopic polyangiitis (MPA). ANCAs are not typically associated with the development of neutropenia. It should be kept in mind that drug induced secondary autoimmune neutropenia (AIN) results from pathogenic antibodies directed against auto-antigens on the neutrophil membrane, or possibly antibodies against membrane antigens expressed on immature granulocyte precursors [44]. Grayson *et al.* addressed the association between ANCA and neutropenia and found 74 patients in the medical literature as of October 2010 [45]. A good number of these patients (24 of 74) were noted to have a drug or toxin related exposure, with the majority having been exposed to either PTU or levamisole. Others were exposed to methimazole, hydralazine, or minocycline. An argument for a direct causal relationship between the presence of ANCA and neutropenia could not be made, as anti-neutrophil membrane antibodies are not commonly assayed and could be just coexistence in the reported cases. A possible exception to the general requirement that drug/toxin induced secondary AIN requires the presence of neutrophil membrane specific antibodies came in the finding of two patients diagnosed with cyclic neutropenia with positive ANCA, and negative MPO/PR3. The patients' sera reacted to a novel cytoplasmic 60 kDa protein that its identity is uncertain. However, the authors speculated that its identity could be human neutrophil elastase (HNE) which is the mutated product in children with cyclic neutropenia [46].

Drug Induced ANCA Associated Vasculitis (AAV)

A number of medications have been implicated in causing drug induced AAV. PTU is the most common reported medication, although some biologic agents particularly TNFα inhibitors are increasing in recognition as culprits as well [47]. Patients with PTU-associated AAV are positive for ANCA, and anti-MPO or anti-PR3. Clinical symptoms may be mild, and may be associated with fever, malaise, arthralgia or myalgia, cutaneous vasculitis, to organ involvement exactly in the fashion of primary AAV [47]. Both rapidly progressive glomerulonephritis and hemoptysis, acute respiratory syndrome, to interstitial pneumonitis had been reported in PTU associated AAV. The question of whether levamisole-cocaine induced cutaneous vasculitis with neutropenia is a form of drug induced AAV may only be a matter of distinction. Unlike PTU or other toxins associated with AAV, significant systemic vasculitis affecting end organs had not been widely reported in levamisole-cocaine cases. However, these observations may change as more cases are described.

Clinical Features and Treatment of Levamisole-Cocaine Vasculopathy

The syndrome of cocaine-levamisole-induced cutaneous vasculitis and associated neutropenia can be suspected based on a tetrad of salient clinical findings. These include neutropenia defined as an absolute neutrophil count (ANC) less than 1500 cells/μL, arthralgia, cutaneous vasculitis, and positive ANCA serologies (Table 1). Patients generally present with extensive skin lesions, from petechiae, to retiform purpura, ulcerations, skin necrosis, to large painful hemorrhagic bullous lesions (Figure 1). An interesting finding that has been consistently reported is a predilection for the involvement of the pinna similar to patients with levamisole induced vasculitis. However, the skin lesions can affect many parts of the body, including abdomen, chest, lower back, scrotum, buttocks, legs, and hands. A general sense of malaise and fever may be present. Skin pathology findings show a small vessel vasculopathy, with a mixed pattern of occlusive thrombosis with varying degrees of small vessel perivascular infiltrates to vasculitis and leukocytoclastic lesions (Figure 2) [49, 48 -51, 50]. Immune complexes with IgM, IgA, IgG and C3 deposition may present in some cases [51]. Treatment of levamisole-cocaine vasculopathy associated skin lesions depends on the extent of body involvement. For petechiae and retiform purpura, oral NSAIDs, oral colchicine, or fixed courses of oral corticosteroids may be appropriate. Disease course after stoppage of levamisole-cocaine had repeatedly been changed dramatically, and skin vasculitis almost always recurred after levamisole-cocaine reuse. For large skin lesions and hemorrhagic bullae leading to skin necrosis, specialized wound and burn care with consideration for autografts may be required [49, 52]. Concurrent agranulocytosis presents a secondary challenge. Empiric antibiotic treatment of neutropenic fever prophylaxis as well as empiric treatment for suspected secondary skin infection may be part of the management particularly in patients with extensive lesions. The exact pathogenesis for skin lesions is unclear, but one may speculate that levamisole induced vasculitis could be amplified by the vasospastic, prothrombotic, and vasculitic effects of cocaine.

Table 1. Clinical Presentations of Cocaine-Levamisole-Induced Vasculopathy and Neutropenia[1]

Age/ Sex/ Route of use	Clinical Signs and Symptoms	Neutropenia	Serologies	Skin Biopsy
57F	Tender purpuric plaques on cheeks and ear lobes,	ANC = 500 cells/μL	pANCA IgM-ACL+	Organizing thrombi in small vessels with perivascular lymphocytic infiltrates
22F	Erythematous plaques with central necrosis on thighs, lower extremities, buttocks and cheeks	ANC < 1000 cells/μL	pANCA IgM-ACL+ Low C3, C4, protein C&S	Small vessel vasculitis with multiple intravascular thrombi
NS/M	Purple discoloration on left upper arm, right second toe and bilateral necrosis of ears	ANC = 1900 cells/μL	Not reported	Not done
39F	Retiform purpura legs and trunk; hemorrhagic bullae legs, trunks, buttocks	No	pANCA, cANCA ANA, LAC Anti-HNE	Microvascular thrombosis with thrombin and recanalization; LCV without thrombosis
49F	Retiform purpura lower limbs, chest, nasal ulcers; leukopenia, lymphopenia,	WBC = 2000 cells/μL ANC = 400 cells/μL	pANCA, cANCA ANA, LAC Anti-HNE, Low MPO, Low PR3	Microvascular thrombosis in dermis and subcutis, fibrinous intraluminal plugs, fibrotic cribriform pattern
38F	Retiform pupura with stellate purpura on ears, cheeks, breast, all extremities	ANC = 550 cells/μL	cANCA LAC, PR3	LCV with mural fibrin depostion, neutrophilic infiltrate, nuclear dust and extravasated erythrocytes with luminal thrombosis in few vessels
43F	stellate purpuric patches and plaques on lower extremities, pinna involved, livedo racemosa	ANC = 560 cells/μL	pANCA, cANCA LAC, IgM-ACL dsDNA, MPO	Occlusion of small superficial and deep dermal blood vessels by fibrin thrombi without vasculitis

Age/ Sex/ Route of use	Clinical Signs and Symptoms	Neutropenia	Serologies	Skin Biopsy
43F	Mottled reticular erythematous patches on lower extremities with scattered punched-out ulcers with central eschars	none	pANCA	Extensive vascular thrombosis
41F	Retiform pupuric patches bilateral thighs, buttocks, trunk, upper extremities, nasal tip	None	pANCA, PR3	Thrombotic vasculopathy

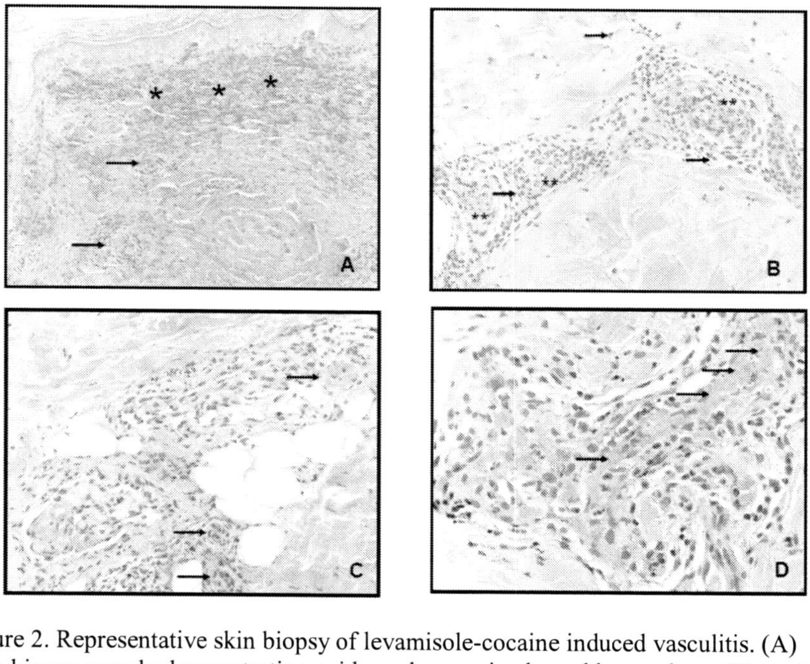

Figure 2. Representative skin biopsy of levamisole-cocaine induced vasculitis. (A) Skin biopsy sample demonstrating epidermal necrosis, dermal hemorrhage (*), and vascular occlusion with fibrin thrombi (arrow) and focal vascular destruction with mild perivascular lymphocytic infiltrate with few neutrophils. (B) Vaso-occlusion with intra-luminal fibrin thrombi (**) and surrounding neutrophilic inflammation with occasional eosinophils (arrow heads). (C) Occlusion and intravascular endothelial proliferation and fibrin deposition within small vessels (arrow). (D) High power showing acute occlusion from exuberant fibrin deposition (arrow) and early intravascular endothelial hyperplasia (hematoxylin and eosin stained); original magnification, x10 (A); x20 (B); x30 (C); and x40 (D).

Not all patients with levamisole-cocaine induced vasculopathy present with agranulocytosis. We and others have seen patients who present with only severe agranulocytosis, while there are patients who may present with only skin manifestations with or without musculoskeletal or other constitutional complaints. The hematologic profile of this syndrome closely mimics those described in levamisole related agranulocytosis, casting the hypothesis that levamisole is the likely component for causing neutropenia especially since cocaine is not a known of agranulocytosis [27]. Anemia, thrombocytopenia, or associated monocytosis are not commonly encountered features. In one study, bone marrow aspirates were notable for granulocytic hypoplasia in 9 out of 13 cocaine-exposed patients. Antineutrophil cytoplasmic antibodies were positive in 3 out of 5 cocaine associated neutropenic patients [27]. ANC nadir was remarkable, and ranging from $0x10^9$ /L to $0.3x10^9$ /L. Relapse of neutropenia again is expected with recurrent levamisole-cocaine exposure [27]. Similar to other forms of drug induced neutropenia, supportive care with antibiotics is the main treatment modality. Granulocyte colony-stimulating factor (GCSF) may be helpful in some selected patients with severe neutropenia (ANC <500 cells/μL) [27, 53].

There is no specific laboratory workup to confirm levamisole-cocaine induced vasculopathy, but a definite pattern has emerged. Confirmation of cocaine exposure by urinary testing and searching for levamisole by gas chromatography/mass spectrometry may provide helpful evidences. Serologically, patients typically have high titers of ANCAs, with a predominance of perinuclear pattern although cytoplasmic pattern can be seen. Specific AAV antigens like PR3 or MPO are seldom positive. In fact, MPO is notably absent or present only in low titers [48, 49, and 54]. Consistent with the idea that levamisole-cocaine induced vasculopathy should be classified as a drug-induced AAV, ANCAs in perinuclear pattern with recognition of other atypical cytoplasmic neutrophil antigens such as lactoferrin, human neutrophil elastase (HNE), and cathepsin G are detected in a case series [47, 48]. ANA, lupus anticoagulant (LAC), IgM anticardiolipin, and IgM anti-β2 glycoprotein antibodies are some other notable serologic markers that can be positive in levamisole-cocaine induced vasculopathy [48, 49].

Vague constitutional symptoms such as malaise, low grade fever and diffuse arthralgia or arthritis affecting the large joints were observed in reported cases of levamisole-cocaine induced vasculopathy. These symptoms can be effectively managed with oral NSAIDs or low dose corticosteroids. Oral or nasal mucosal lesions were also observed perhaps owing to local trauma by the route of cocaine use. From March 2009 to November 2010,

McGrath *et al.* performed a retrospective study of thirty ANCA positive cases with associated cocaine use at Massachusetts General Hospital to further delineate patients with levamisole-cocaine vasculopathy. They reaffirmed the finding that skin lesions (61%) and arthralgia/arthritis (83%) were the most presentation [55]. Fever, malaise, weight loss, and myalgias were also reported. Abnormal urinalysis, defined as dipstick proteinuria, hematuria, or cellular/RBC casts on microscopy also reported in 8 out of 30 patients by authors. Two patients developed severe acute kidney injury with active urine sediment [55]. One patient was found to have pauci-immune focal necrotizing and crecentic glomerulonephritis (GN). Both patients required treatment with immunosuppressive agents, and ultimately required renal replacement therapy. Pulmonary hemorrhage was also observed in three different patients in this cohort, but none required intubation. A worthwhile distinction in this cohort was the finding of positive anti-MPO in four individuals with biopsy proven vasculitis, including a case of pauci-immune GN, which differed from prior observations.

Conclusion

A novel syndrome of levamisole-cocaine induced vasculopathy and neutropenia is increasingly seen in clinical practice owing to the prevalence of illicit cocaine use. The immunomodulatory properties of levamisole and the vasospastic, thrombotic, and vasculitic features of cocaine provide the underpinning for this unique syndrome. Since its recognition, the majority of patients presented with severe neutropenia alone or in combination with extensive skin lesions in the absence of significant organ involvement. Serologic testing usually reveals high ANCA titer with perinuclear or cytoplasmic patterns, positive ANA, and lupus anticoagulant or anticardiolipin antibodies. IgM or IgG anti-neutrophil antibodies are useful markers to identify levamisole-induced AIN. Nevertheless, the clinical spectrum of levamisole-cocaine induced vasculopathy may be evolving and becoming reminiscent of more "typical" drug induced AAV cases the same as patients with PTU induced AAV. Renal and pulmonary involvement had already been described in a retrospective cohort. Longitudinal observation of future patients will determine if the spectrum of disease may be more encompassing than already known.

References

[1] Centers for Disease Control and prevention (CDC). Agranulocytosis associated with cocaine use — four states, March 2008-November 2009. *MMWR Morb. Mortal Wkly Rep.,* 2009;58:1381-5.

[2] Thompson, J. S., Herbick J. M., Vogel, C. L. Studies on Levamisole - Induced Agranulocytosis. *Blood,* 1980;56:388-396.

[3] Moertel C. G., Fleming T. R., Macdonald J. S., Haller D. G., Laurie J. A., Goodman P. J. Levamisole and Fluorouracil for adjuvant therapy of resected colon carcinoma. *N. Engl. J. Med.,* 1990; 322:352-358.

[4] Veys E. M., Mielants H., Verbruggen G. Gold salts, levamisole and D-penicillamine as first choice slow-acting antirheumatic drugs in rheumatoid arthritis – a long-term follow-up study. *Clin. Exp. Rheumatol.*, 1987;5:111-116.

[5] Chang A., Osterloh J., Thomas J. Levamisole: A dangerous new cocaine adulterant. *Clin. Pharmacol. Ther.*, 2010;88:408-411.

[6] Knowles L., Buxton J. A., Skuridina N., Achebe I., LeGatt D., Fan S., Zhu N. Y., Talbot J. Levamisole tainted cocaine causing severe neutropenia in Alberta and British Columbia. *Harm. Reduct. J.,* 2009;6:30.

[7] Thienpont D., Vanparijs O. F. J., Raeymaekers A. H. M., Vandenberk J., Demoen P. J. A., Allewijn F. T. N., et al. Tetramisole (R 8299), a new, potent broad spectrum anthelmintic. *Nature,* 1966;209:1084 – 1086.

[8] Martin, R. J., Roberson A. P. Mode of action of levamisole and pyrantel, anthelmintic resistance, E153 and Q57. *Parasitology*, 2007:134;1093-1104.

[9] Albonico M., Bickle Q., Ramsan M., Montresor A., Savioli L., Taylor M. Efficacy of mebendazole and levamisole alone or in combination against intestinal nematode infections after repeated targeted mebendazole treatment in Zanzibar. *Bull. World Health Organ.,* 2003; 81:343-352.

[10] Lombel R. M., Gipson D. S., Hodson, E. M. Treatment of steroid-sensitive nephrotic syndrome: new guidelines from KDIGO. *Pediatr. Nephrol.*, 2013;28:415-426.

[11] Hodson E. M., Willis N. S., Craig J. C. Non-corticosteroid treatment for nephrotic syndrome in children. *Cochrane Database Syst. Rev.,* 2008 Jan. 23;(1):CD002290.

[12] Williams, G. T., Johnson S. A., Huskinsson E. C., et al. Neutropenia during treatment of rheumatoid arthritis with levamisole. *Ann. Rheum. Dis.,* 1978;37:366-369.

[13] Runge L. A., Pinals R. S., Lourie S. H., Tomar R. H. Treatment of rheumatoid arthritis with levamisole. A controlled trial. *Arthritis Rheum.,* 1977;20:1445-1448.

[14] Runge L. A., Pinals R. S., Tomar R. H. Treatment of rheumatoid arthritis with levamisole: long-term results and immune changes. *Ann. Rheum. Dis.,* 1979;38:122-127.

[15] Mowat A.G. Neutrophil chemotaxis in rheumatoid arthritis. *Annals of the Rheumatic Diseases,* 1978; 37: 1-8

[16] QUASAR Collaborative Group. Adjuvant chemotherapy versus observation in patients with colorectal cancer: a randomised study. *Lancet,* 2007;370: 2020–2029.

[17] Sajid M. S., Iqbal Z., Icqbal M. U. Immunomodulatory effect of various anti-parasitics: a review. *Parasitology,* 2006:132:301-313.

[18] Smahel M., Polakova I., Vajdova E. Systemic adminstration of CpG Oligodeoxynucleotide and levamisole as adjuvants for gene-gun-delivered anti-tumor DNA vaccines. *Clin. Dev. Immunol.*, 2011: Epub. 2011 Oct. 18.

[19] Mitchell M. S. Combinations of anticancer drugs and immunotherapy. *Cancer Immunol. Immunother.*, 2003:52;686-692.

[20] Alavian S. M., Tabatabaei S. V. The effect of diabetes mellitus on immunological response to hepatitis B virus vaccine in individuals with chronic kidney disease: A meta-analysis of current literature. *Vaccine,* 2010;28:3773-3777.

[21] Davin J. C., Merkus M. P. Levamisole in steroid-sensitive nephrotic syndrome of childhood: the lost paradise? *Pediatr. Nephrol.*, 2005; 20: 10-14.

[22] Goldin A., Chirigos M. A., Mihich E. Biologic response modifiers and adjuvant chemoherapy: consideration of selected preclinical investigations in relation to clinical potential. *Recent Results Cancer Res.,* 1982: 80,351-356.

[23] Levandoski M. M., Piket B., Chang J. The anthelminthic levamisole is an allosteric modulator of human neuronal nicotinic acetylcholine receptors. *Eur. J. Pharmacol.*, 2003; 471:9-20.

[24] Larocque A., Hoffman R. S. Levamisole in cocaine: Unexpected news from an old acquaintance. *Clin. Toxicol. (Phila.),* 2012; 50:231-241.

[25] Francis, M. M., Vazquez, R. W., Oswald, R. E. Subtype-Selective Inhibition of Neuronal Nicotinic Acetylcholine Receptors by Cocaine Is Determined by the a4 and b4 Subunits. *Mol. Pharmacol.*, 2000; 58: 109-119.

[26] Veys E. M., Mielants H., Verbruggen G. Levamisole-induced adverse reactions in HLA B27-positive rheumatoid arthritis. *Lancet,* 1978; 1:148.

[27] Czuchlewski D. R., Brackney M., Faucar K. Clinicopathologic Features of Agranulocytosis in the Setting of Levamisole-Tainted Cocaine. *Am. J. Clin. Pathol.,* 2010; 133:466-472.

[28] Thompson J. S., Herbick J. M., Vogel C. L. et. al. Studies on levamisole--induced agranulocytosis. *Blood,* 1980; 56:388-96.

[29] Macfarlane D. G., Bacon P. A. Levamisole-induced vasculitis due to circulating immune complexes. *Br. Med. J.,* 1978;1:407-408.

[30] Bagga A., Hari P. Levamisole-induced vasculitis. *Pediatr. Nephrol.,* 2000; 14:1057-1058.

[31] Barbano G., Ginevri F., Ghiggeri G. M., Gusmano R. Disseminated autoimmune disease during levamisole treatment of nephrotic syndrome. *Pediatr. Nephrol.,* 1999;13:602-603.

[32] Laux-End R., Inaebnit D., Gerber H. A., Bianchetti M. G. Vasculitis associated with levamisole and circulating autoantibodies. *Arch. Dis. Child.,* 1996; 75:355-356.

[33] Menni S., Pistritto G., Gianotti R., Ghio L., Edefonti A. Ear lobe bilateral necrosis by levamisole-induced occlusive vasculitis in a pediatric patient. *Pediatr. Dermatol.,* 1997; 14:477-9.

[34] Rongioletti F., Ghio L., Ginevri F., Bleidl D., Rinaldi S., Edefonti A. et al. Purpura of the ears: a distinctive vasculopathy with circulating autoantibodies complicating long-term treatment with levamisole in children. *Br. J. Dermatol.,* 1999; 140:948-951.

[35] Brewer, J. D., Meves, A., Pittelkow M. R. Cocaine abuse: Dermatologic manifestations and therapeutic approaches. *J. Am. Acad. Dermatol.,* 2008; 59:483-487.

[36] Orriols R., Munoz X., Morell. Cocaine-induced Churg-Strauss vasculitis. *Eur. Respir. J.,* 1996; 9:175–177.

[37] Neynaber, S., Mistry-Burchardi, N., Wollenberg A., et al. PR3-ANCA-positive Necrotizing Multi-organ Vasculitis Following Cocaine Abuse. *Acta. Derm. Venereol.*, 2008; 88:594–596.

[38] Merkel, P. A., Koroshetz, W. J., Cudkowicz, M. E., et al. Cocaine-Associated Cerebral Vasculitis. *Semin. Arthritis Rheum.*, 1995; 25:172-183.

[39] Friedman D. R., Wolfsthal, S. D. Cocaine-induced pseudovasculitis. *Mayo Clin. Proc.*, 2005; 80:671-673.

[40] Hofbauer G. F., Hafner, J., Trueb, R. M. Urticarial vasculitis following cocaine use. *Br. J. Dermat.*, 1999: 141: 600-6001.

[41] Wiesner O., Russell K. A., Lee A. S., Jenne D. E., Trimarchi M., Gregorini G. et al. Antineutrophil cytoplasmic antibodies reacting with human neutrophil elastase as a diagnostic marker for cocaine-induced midline destructive lesions but not autoimmune vasculitis. *Arthritis Rheum.*, 2004; 50:2954-2965.

[42] Trimarchi M., Gregorini G., Facchetti F., et al. Cocaine-induced midlined destructive lesions: clinical, radiographic, histopathologic, and serologic features and their differentiation from Wegener granulomatosis. *Medicine (Baltimore),* 2001; 80:391–404.

[43] Stahelin L., Fialho S. C., Pereira I. A., et al. Cocaine-induced midline destruction lesions with positive ANCA test mimicking Wegener's granulomatosis. *Rev. Bras. Reumatol.*, 2012; 52:431-437.

[44] Newman, K. A., Akhtari M. Management of autoimmune neutropenia in Felty's syndrome and systemic lupus erythematosus. *Autoimmun. Rev.,* 2011; 10:432-437.

[45] Grayson, P. C., Slone, M. J., Merkel P. A., et al. Antineutrophil Cytoplasmic Antibodies, Autoimmune Neutropenia, and Vasculitis. *Semin. Arthritis Rheum.*, 2011: 41:424-433.

[46] Rodrigues, C. E., Velloso, E. R., Carvalho J. F. A novel 60 kDa reactivity in cyclic neutropenia: High titer cytoplasmic ANCA immunostaining pattern and negative anti-proteinase-3 antibody. *Joint Bone Spine*, 2011; 78:319–325.

[47] Gao, Y., Zhao, M. H. Review article: Drug-induced anti-neutrophil cytoplasmic antibody-associated vasculitis. *Nephrology (Carlton),* 2009; 14,: 33–41.

[48] Graf, J., Lynch, K., Imboden J., et al. Purpura, Cutaneous Necrosis, and Antineutrophil Cytoplasmic Antibodies Associated With Levamisole-Adulterated Cocaine. *Arthritis and Rheumatism*, 2011; 63:3998–4001.

[49] Poon S. H., Baliog C. R., Reginato, A. M. Syndrome of Cocaine-Levamisole Induced Cutaneous Vasculitis and Immune Mediated Leukopenia. *Semin. Arthritis Rheum.*, 2011; 41:434-44.

[50] Espinosa L. R., Alamino R. P. Cocaine-Induced Vasculitis: Clinical and Immunological Spectrum. *Curr. Rheumatol. Rep.,* 2012; 14:532–538.

[51] Lee, K. C., Ladizinski B., Federman, D. G. Complications Associated With Use ofLevamisole-Contaminated Cocaine: An Emerging Public Health Challenge. *Mayo Clin. Proc.,* 2012; 87:581–586.

[52] Ching J. A., Smith D. J. Jr. Levamisole-induced necrosis of skin, soft tissue, and bone: case report and review of literature. *J. Burn Care Res.,* 2012; 33:e1-5.

[53] Andersohn, F., Konzen, C., Garbe, E. Systematic Review: Agranulocytosis Induced by Nonchemotherapy Drugs. *Ann. Intern. Med.,* 2007; 146:657-665.

[54] Graf, J. Rheumatic manifestations of cocaine use. *Curr. Opin. Rheumatol.,* 2013; 25:50–55.

[55] McGrath M. M., Isakova T., Niles, J. L. Contaminated Cocaine and Antineutrophil Cytoplasmic Antibody-Associated Disease. *Clin. J. Am. Soc. Nephrol.*, 2011; 6: 2799–2805.

[56] Arora, N. P. Cutaneous Vasculopathy and Neutropenia Associated With Levimasole-Adulterated Cocaine. *The American Journal of the Medical Sciences,* 2013; 345: 45-50.

In: Neutropenia
Editors: M. Akhtari et al.
ISBN: 978-1-63482-105-6

Chapter 7

Pulmonary and Critical Care Considerations in Neutropenic Patients

Indryas Woldie[1] and Ayman O. Soubani[2]
[1]Department of Oncology, Karmanos Cancer Center
and Wayne State University School of Medicine, Wayne State University,
School of Medicine, Detroit, MI, US
[2]Pulmonary and Critical Care Service,
Karmanos Cancer Center and Wayne State University School of Medicine,
Wayne State University School of Medicine, Detroit, MI, US

Introduction

Definition and Classification

Neutrophils are the final cells in the maturation of granulocytes and have significant role in defense against infection. Neutropenia is generally defined as absolute neutrophile count (ANC) ≤ 1500/mm^3 in adults. Neutropenia can be classified to mild without increased risk of infections, and severe to profound with increased predisposition to infections (Table 1). Risk of infection is usually increased when the ANC falls below 500/ mm^3. However, there are additional important host and microbial factors that determine whether patients will actually develop infection despite neutropenia [1].

Etiology

Neutropenia can be classified as acquired versus congenital (Table 2). Chemotherapeutic agents have variable bone marrow suppressive effect. In addition, combination of myelo-suppressive agents, age, patient co-morbidities and presence of underlying bone marrow disease play major role in development of neutropenia. High dose chemotherapy prior to autologous stem cell transplant and preparative regimen prior to allogeneic hematopoietic stem cell transplant are always followed by a period of neutropenia. Infections and in particular viral infections can suppress bone marrow and result in neutropenia. HIV, hepatitis B and C, and cytomegalovirus (CMV) are the usual culprits, and particularly in an immune-compromised host can be a long list. There is a long list of medications that may cause neutropenia. In a population-based, case-cohort study antithyroid drugs, trimethoprim-sulfamethoxazole, sulfasalazine, clomipramine, and dipyrone combined with analgesics had the strongest relative risk with severe drug induced neutropenia [2].

Consequences of neutropenia including a variety of infectious and non-infectious complications involve several organs in the body. This chapter will focus on pulmonary and critical care considerations in management of neutropenia secondary to chemotherapy and/or stem cell transplantation. We will review the main conditions that lead to critical illness in neutropenic patients and suggest an approach to diagnosis and management of these conditions.

Neutropenic Fever

Neutropenic fever is a serious medical condition that if it is not treated promptly can be fatal. Neutropenic fever defined as oral temperature of $\geq 38.3^0$ Celsius (101^0F) in a patient with ANC of $\leq 500/mm^3$[3].

In 10-50% of patients with solid tumors and up to 80% of patients with hematologic malignancy fever may complicate chemotherapy with inducing neutropenia. Nevertheless, no infectious agent can be found in up to 70% of patients [4-5].

Table 1. Classification of Neutropenia

Degree	Mild	Moderate	Severe	Profound
ANC/mm^3	1000-1500	500-1000	< 500	< 100

Table 2. Etiologies of Neutropenia

- Acquired:
  - Drug Induced Bone Marrow Suppression
    - Chemotherapeutic agents
    - Antiviral agents (Ganciclovir)
    - Antipsychotics
    - Antithyroid drugs, Trimethoprim-Sulfamethoxazole, Sulfasalazine, Clomipramine, Others.
  - Autoimmune
    - Systemic Lupus Erythematosus
    - Rheumatoid Arthritis
    - Drug Induced
  - Infections
    - Viral (HIV, Hepatitis, CMV)
    - Bacterial
    - Parasitic infections
  - Bone marrow failure
    - Acute Leukemia
    - Myelodysplastic syndrome
    - Myelofibrosis
    - Aplastic anemia
  - Nutritional
    - Vitamin B 12 deficiency
    - Copper deficiency
- Congenital:
  - Cyclic Neutropenia
  - Severe Congenital Neutropenia
  - Fanconi Syndrome
  - Others

Both gram negative and gram positive organisms can complicate neutropenia. Mucositis secondary to chemotherapy and widespread use of central venous catheters provide portal of infection. The most common sites of infection in neutropenic patients and underlying malignancy are gastrointestinal tract, lung and skin [4].

In a retrospective study, chemotherapy-associated FN patients who received care in ED reviewed [6]. In this study only 9% of patients had possible identifiable source of infection and rate of bacteremia in cancer patients with neutropenic fever was as high as 37% [6]. Gram positive organisms are also important culprits as skin and catheter associated infections complicate neutropenia. Recent evidence suggests gram positive organisms are becoming more common in neutropenic patients. In addition, significant proportion of infections in neutropenic patients can be polymicrobial [7].

Patients with neutropenic fever who are admitted to critical care unit are seriously ill owing to evidence of end organ damage including but not limited to hypotension unresponsive to fluid boluses, altered level of consciousness, respiratory failure, and disseminated intravascular coagulation. Timely management is very critical, and early and appropriate intervention determines outcome in these critically ill patients.

Management of neutropenic fever in intensive care unit comprises stabilization and supportive care, empiric antimicrobial therapy, appropriate laboratory and imaging work up and timely interpretation and decision making (Figure 1).

Physical exam in patients with neutropenic fever should be focused on potential sites of infection including skin and mucus membrane, catheter sites, lung, abdomen and inspection of perianal area. Rectal exam should be avoided in neutropenic patients as it may result in tissue injury and introduction of bacteria in to the blood stream.

Initial work up of patients with febrile neutropenia (FN) is likely to be completed prior to admission to intensive care unit. In addition to a good history and focused physical exam, complete blood count with differential, comprehensive metabolic profile (with renal and liver function tests), urinalysis with or without culture, lactic acid level, blood cultures from central and peripheral sites and appropriate imaging should be done. Furthermore, as guided by clinical history and physical findings, additional cultures, imaging and laboratory data including CT chest/abdomen and sinuses, serum galactomannan antigen, urine legionella, pneumococcal and histoplasma antigen may be needed. In patients with persistently positive blood cultures and fungemia, echocardiogram should be obtained to rule out endocarditis [4].

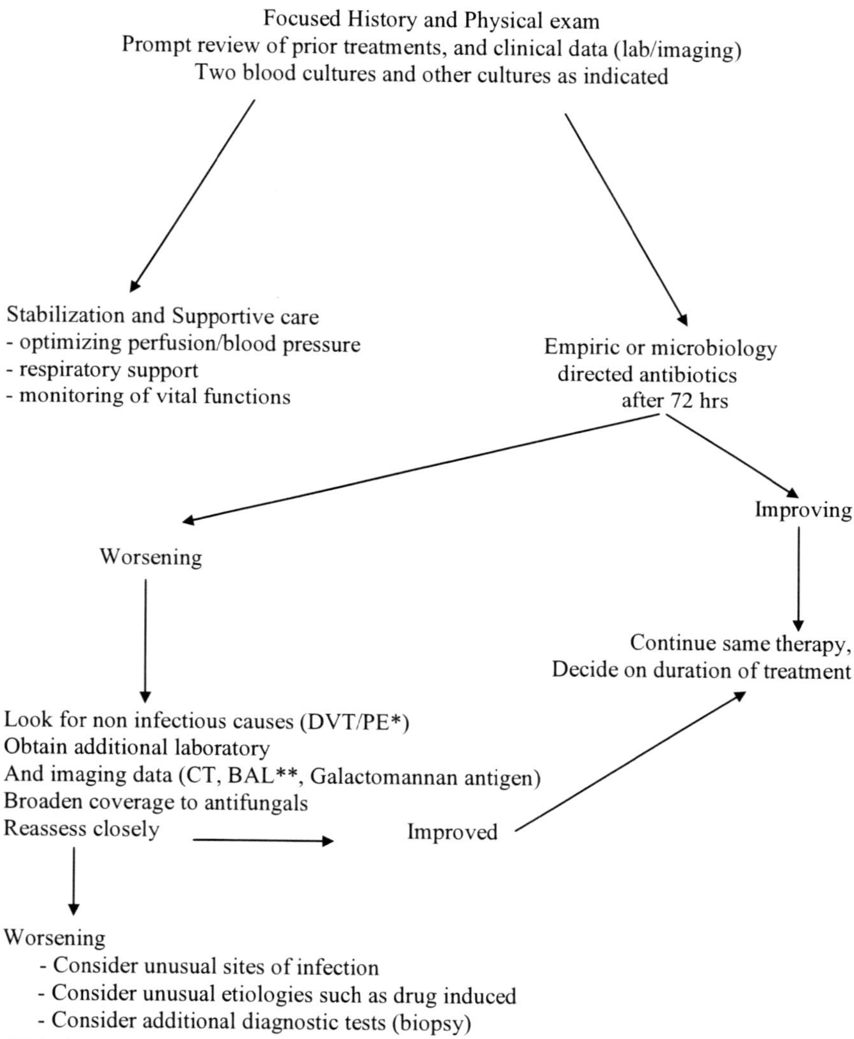

* DVT: deep venous thrombosis. PE: pulmonary embolism.
** BAL: broncho-alveolar lavage.

Figure 1. Approach to patients with febrile neutropenia who are admitted to pulmonary and critical care unit.

High resolution chest CT scan, bronchoscopy with bronchoalveolar lavage (BAL), and occasionally lung biopsy are reserved for patients suspected of having respiratory infection and not clinically improving. In addition to the commonly ordered aerobic and anaerobic cultures, sample from patients who had BAL should be sent for a viral, fungal and mycobacterial studies, pneumocystis stain and serological fungal tests such as (1→3)-β-D-glucan and aspergillus galactomannan antigen [3].

Treatment of Febrile Neutropenia

After stabilization of patient and getting adequate measures of hemodynamic parameters, treatment of febrile neutropenia requires prompt decision making and initiation of both empiric and microbiology directed therapy. The initial empiric treatment for chemotherapy induced febrile neutropenia in hemodynamically stable patients is monotherapy with a beta-lactam such as cefepime, a carbapenem (imipenem, meropenem) or piperacillin-tazobactam to cover pseudomonas species. For patients who are hemodynamically unstable with hypotension, those with suspected pneumonia or those who failed to respond to the initial monotherapy regimen, additional agents including vancomycin, aminoglycosides and fluoroquinolones should be considered [4, 8]. In addition, local microbial resistance patterns should be taken into consideration when making a decision on empiric antibiotic coverage.

A prospective study on 255 patients in Japan showed that monotherapy with either carbapenem or cefepime as initial agent in patients with febrile neutropenia have the same efficacy. The same study also demonstrated that in patients who failed to respond to first line therapy, aminoglycosides and ciprofloxacin have comparable efficacy as a second line agents [5]. In a randomized, double blind multi-center study linezolid was compared to vancomycin in patients with febrile neutropenia due to gram positive organisms. This study demonstrated that linezolid has the same efficacy and safety profile as vancomycin in patients with FN [9].

Daptomycin is a lipopeptide antibiotic which is rapidly bacteriocidal against gram positive bacteria. It is an effective alternative in patients with methicillin-resistant Staphylococcus aureus (MRSA) with reduced susceptibility to vancomycin and in cases of vancomycin resistant enterococcus [7].

Patients with profound and prolonged neutropenia for more than 7 days are at high risk for invasive fungal infections. Additional risk factors for invasive fungal infection in intensive care unit include advanced age, central venous catheters, broad spectrum antibiotic use, total parenteral nutrition, hematologic malignancy and renal failure. Empiric antifungal therapy should be started in neutropenic patients who are still febrile after 72 hours of antibiotics. The choice of specific agent should be based on previous use of prophylactic antifungal and patient specific clinical picture. Initial empiric antifungal agents include caspofungin followed by liposomal amphotericin B. In case of aspergillus infection, voriconazole is the preferred agent [10].

In a multicenter, open-labeled, randomized trial, empiric antifungal therapy for persistent or recurrent fever compared with pre-emptive antifungal therapy for treatment of patients who have clinical, imaging and laboratory assay, specifically galactomannan antigen, suggestive of fungal disease. This study revealed higher incidence of invasive fungal disease in the pre-emptive group without increasing mortality [11].

Currently, empiric antifungal therapy is the standard of care for neutropenic patients who continue to be febrile after few days of antimicrobial therapy [12].

Severe Sepsis

Sepsis is a systemic response to infection. It is a syndrome which comprises the presence of systemic inflammatory response (SIRS) and possible focus of infection. SIRS includes signs and symptoms of tachycardia, tachypnea, fever or hypothermia and leukocytosis or leukopenia. It is called severe sepsis when sepsis is complicated with end organ dysfunction such as hypotension, respiratory failure, altered mental status, disseminated intravascular coagulation, and carries a very high risk of mortality [13].

Sepsis in neutropenic patients requires particular attention as its course and presentation may be different for several reasons. Typical manifestations of infection may not be seen as the main mediators of infection, neutrophils, are missing. In addition, infections from otherwise uncommon organisms may occur and should be suspected in neutropenic patients. The clinical course of sepsis in neutropenic patients who also have additional causes of compromised immunity may be rapidly progressive. Thus, early admission and care in intensive care unit is mandatory for all neutropenic patients with sepsis that show signs of end organ dysfunction.

A retrospective study of 102 neutropenic patients demonstrated that neutropenic patients with sepsis and underlying malignancy have 58% of 30 day mortality. This study also showed that presence of organ failure is a significant determinant of 30 day mortality, and emphasizing the need to prevent development of organ failure [14].

In a retrospective study from 1998 to 2008, survival of 428 intensive care unit patients with cancer, neutropenia, and severe sepsis or septic shock reviewed. This study revealed that patients' survival increased over this period showing importance of early antibiotic therapy. However, mortality was as high as 43% and the same as non-neutropenic non-cancer patients in recent reports. The survival was higher in patients who admitted to ICU as early as possible. Older age, need for vasopressors, neurologic, respiratory or hepatic dysfunction and acute noninfectious conditions were independent predicted factors for higher mortality in this study. On the other hand admission to the intensive care unit after 2003, combination antibiotic therapy including an aminoglycoside, and early indwelling catheter removal were associated with reduced mortality [15].

Early Goal Directed Therapy (EGDT)

In a retrospective case series study, early goal-oriented therapy EGDT, corticosteroid administration, and rhAPC administration have been shown to be an effective tool in avoiding treatment delay and reducing mortality in patients with sepsis. Initiation of antibiotics, fluid resuscitation and respiratory support are major areas of delay in treatment of sepsis that affect outcome [16].

Quick assessment and triage of patients as well as adequate fluid resuscitation are the major components of EGDT. Mean arterial pressure > 65 mmHg, central venous pressure 8-12 cmH2O, urine output > 0.5 ml/kg/hr and central venous oxygen saturation > 70% are therapeutic goals in resuscitation of these patients. EGDT may be achieved by starting intravenous fluids immediately in form of crystalloid such as normal saline. In the condition patient remains hypotensive or has low serum albumin, then albumin may be added. If central venous oxygen saturation remains low despite of adequate fluid resuscitation, transfusing of packed red blood cells in patients with low hemoglobin or adding dobutamine to increase cardiac output may improve oxygen delivery to tissues [17]. These patients usually require addition of vasopressors to maintain blood pressure. Norepinephrine has been shown to be the best vasopressor agent in patients with severe sepsis or septic shock. Dopamine is an alternative and epinephrine or vasopressin may be added if patient remains hypotensive. Initiation of antibiotics in a timely manner after obtaining blood cultures is essential. Every effort should be made to start antibiotics within the first 3 hours of presentation, especially in septic neutropenic patients. There is a strong correlation between death and delay in antibiotics in patients with severe sepsis [18].

Initiation of antimicrobials in a timely manner after obtaining blood culture, hemodynamic monitoring using central venous catheter and arterial line, respiratory support and continuous assessment of response and decision making for additional intervention as needed may improve absolute mortality rate of septic patients. It also important to control the source of infection –such as removal of infected vascular catheter or drainage of an abscess- as soon as possible [19].

In a prospective study of 1177 patients with primary or secondary infection, it has been demonstrated that lactic acid level > or= 4 nmol/l predict a higher mortality in acute phase of patients with sepsis [20]. A retrospective study in an emergency department of a comprehensive cancer center showed that implementation of order set and algorithm for EGDT in patients with severe sepsis was associated with reduced 28 day in hospital mortality rate [21].

Invasive Fungal Infection

Invasive fungal infection (IFI) is one of the complications of prolonged and profound neutropenia that carries very high mortality. In a matched case control study of all solid organ transplant recipients admitted to intensive care unit, 2.7% of patients developed documented invasive fungal infection and case fatality was as high as 60%. Aspergillosis was the commonest etiology followed by candidiasis in this study [22].

Candidiasis

Candida albicans is the most common cause of candidemia, followed by non-albicans species including *C. glabrata, C. parapsilosis, C. tropicalis* and *C. krusei.* Since starting fluconazole prophylaxis for high risk patients, incidence of invasive candidiasis has been significantly reduced. However not all Candida are sensitive to fluconazole and some patients can develop breakthrough candidemia. Risk factors for invasive candidiasis are generally similar to other invasive fungal infections and include prolonged neutropenia, indwelling catheter, total parentral nutrition and use of broad spectrum antibiotics [22].

Positive blood culture for candida fungemia which can be detected on routine blood cultures should not be considered as contamination. Once diagnosed, therapy should be instituted promptly along with removal of indwelling catheters particularly when cultures remain persistently positive. Blood cultures should be done on a daily basis till becomes negative for two consecutive days. Antifungal therapy should be continued for at least 14 days since the last negative blood culture [23].

Fluconazole has excellent activity against *C. albicans* with good safety profile and can be used in non neutropenic patients with candidemia. However, some strains of *C. glabrata* and all strains of *C. Krusei* are resistant to fluconazole. Compared to fluconazole, voriconazole has superior activity against all species of candida except in cases of cross resistance particularly with *C. glabrata*. Echinocandins including micafungin, caspofungin and anidulafungin are effective against most species of candida. Occasionally *C. parapsilosis* and *C. glabrata* may develop resistance. Echinocandins are recommended for most neutropenic patients with candidemia. Fluconazole is a less favored alternative for stable patients with no recent exposure to azoles. In situations where additional coverage is needed for mold infections, voriconazole can be used [24].

Aspergillosis

Invasive aspergillosis (IA) is a serious infection that can be seen in patients with severe and prolonged neutropenia. Additional risk factors for IA include high dose steroid and impaired cellular immunity due to drugs or diseases like AIDS. Patients with marked immunodeficiency, and particularly hematopoietic stem cell transplant and solid organ transplant recipients have the highest incidence of IA justifying prophylactic voriconazole in stem cell transplant patients who are on high dose steroid [25].

Risk of IA will increase steadily with the duration of neutropenia. In a case control study of patients with acute leukemia, risk factors for developing invasive pulmonary aspergillosis were evaluated. The study revealed that risk of developing invasive pulmonary aspergillosis in neutropenic patients will increase by 1% per day for the first 3 weeks and by 4% per day thereafter [26]. In hematopoietic stem cell transplant recipients, allogeneic compared to autologous HSCT has much higher risk of IA with incidence of 2.3-15% and 0.5-4% respectively [27-28].

Diagnosis of invasive pulmonary aspergillosis (IPA) is challenging. Early diagnosis in HSCT recipients remains difficult and high index of suspicion is necessary in patients with risk factors for invasive disease. Histopathological diagnosis by examining lung tissue obtained by thoracoscopic or open lung biopsy remains the "gold standard" for diagnosis of IPA [29]. Presence of septate acute branching hyphae invading the lung tissue along with a positive culture for Aspergillus from the same site is diagnostic for IPA. A retrospective study of autopsy-proven invasive fungal infections (IFI) in patients with hematologic malignancies demonstrated that 77% of IFI were significantly related to patients' death but only one third of them were diagnosed antemortem. In the same study, histopathologic findings of IPA showed a difference depending on the underlying disease. In patients with allogeneic HSCT and GVHD there was intense inflammation and low fungal burden, while in neutropenic patients, IPA was characterized by scant inflammation, extensive coagulation necrosis associated with hyphal angioinvasion, and high fungal burden. Dissemination to other organs was equally high in both groups [30].

Chest radiograph has minor role in early stages of IPA since there is high incidence of non-specific changes. Usual findings include rounded densities, pleural-based infiltrates that are suggestive of pulmonary infarctions, and cavitations. Pleural effusions are uncommon. Multiple inflammatory nodules, often with one large dominant mass are characteristic findings in chest computed tomography [31]. Routine use of chest HRCT early in the course of IPA leads to earlier diagnosis and improved outcome of these patients [32]. Typical chest CT findings include ill defined consolidation (48%), nodules with halo sign (44%), centrilobular nodules (44%), ground glass attenuation (22%), and pleural effusion (26%) (Figure 2) [33]. Halo sign is mainly seen in neutropenic patients early in the course of infection (usually in the first week), and appears as a zone of low attenuation due to hemorrhage surrounding the pulmonary nodule. Air crescent sign, which represents crescent-shaped lucency secondary to necrosis in the region of original nodule is another late radiological sign [31]. Both halo and air crescent signs are neither sensitive nor pathognomonic of IPA.

In HSCT recipients, isolating Aspergillus species from sputum is highly predictive of invasive disease with a positive predictive value of 80-90% [34]. However, negative sputum sample does not rule out IPA [35]. Blood cultures are rarely positive. Bronchoscopy with BAL is generally helpful in diagnosis of IPA, especially in patients with diffuse lung involvement. Sensitivity and specificity of a positive BAL result are 50% and 97% respectively. Yield of positive BAL in diagnosis of IPA is not consistent, and there are reports of much lower diagnostic yield. Transbronchial biopsies usually do not add much to the diagnosis and are associated with increased risk of bleeding, and usually are not suggested [36].

The most recent advances in diagnosis of IPA are related to detecting Aspergillus antigens in body fluids. Galactomannan (GM) is a polysaccharide cell-wall component that is released by Aspergillus during growth. Detection of serum GM by double sandwich ELISA has a threshold of 0.5 ng/ml with 71% sensitivity and 89% specificity, and has been approved by the Food and Drug Administration for diagnosis of IPA [37]. Serum GM may be detected several days before presence of clinical signs, an abnormal chest radiograph, or positive culture. Thus, GM detection may allow earlier confirmation of diagnosis and serial determination of serum GM values may be useful in assessing the evolution of infection during treatment [38].

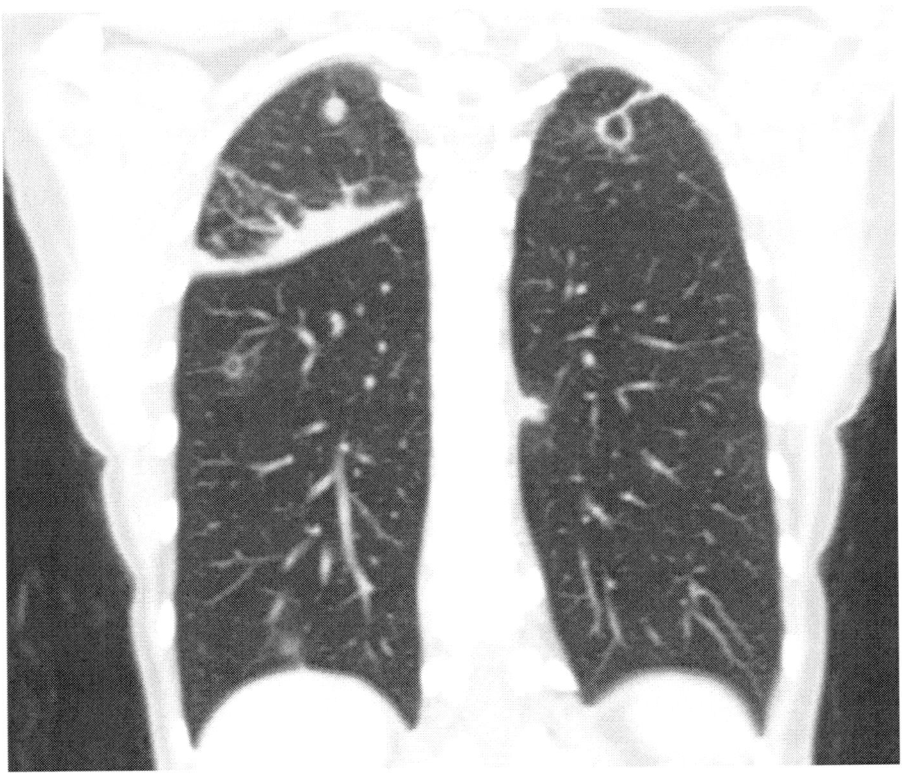

Figure 2. Chest CT image showing bilateral pulmonary nodules, some with cavitation in a neutropenic patient with acute leukemia and invasive aspergillosis.

Serum GM assay is more useful in hematological malignancy patients or allogeneic HSCT recipients than in solid-organ transplant recipients or non-neutropenic patients. Furthermore, BAL Galactomannan assay may add to the sensitivity of serum GM and to other diagnostic methods [39]. In patients with hematologic malignancies and HSCT recipients, sensitivity and specificity of BAL GM in diagnosing proven or probable IPA are 73% and 89% respectively with cutoff of ≥0.5 and 67% and 95% respectively with a cutoff of ≥0.85 [39].

Detection of Aspergillus DNA in BAL fluid and serum by polymerase chain reaction (PCR) is another way to diagnose IPA. A positive Aspergillus PCR in BAL fluid has an estimated sensitivity of 67%-100% and specificity between 55% and 95% [40]. PCR sensitivity and specificity have also been reported at 100% and 65%-92% respectively in serum samples [40]. However, PCR doesn't discriminate between colonization and infection, and often associated with false positive results. Detection of serum (1→3)-β-D-glucan, a fungal cell wall constituent has recently received Food and Drug Administration approval. Determination of plasma (1→3)-β-D-glucan has been reported to be a highly sensitive and specific test for invasive deep mycosis, including candidiasis, fusariosis, and aspergillosis, and could be useful in immunocompromised patients [41]. However, utility of this assay in allogeneic HSCT recipients with high risk of IPA is not yet defined.

Treatment of IPA is difficult and mortality rate is still high despite the introduction of several new antifungal agents. Therapy should be started as soon as there is a clinical suspicion of IPA, and workup is still underway. For many years, amphotericin B has been the first line of therapy for IPA. Recommended dose is 1 to 1.5 mg/kg/day. Amphotericin B is known to cause serious side effects including nephrotoxicity, electrolyte disturbances, and hypersensitivity. Newer lipid-based preparations of amphotericin B such as liposomal amphotericin B and lipid complex amphotericin B have been introduced to reduce the toxicity. Voriconazole is a new broad-spectrum triazole which is approved for initial treatment of invasive aspergillosis, and is currently considered as treatment of choice [36]. Voriconazole is available in both intravenous and oral formulations, and recommended dose is 6 mg/kg twice daily intravenously on day one followed by 4 mg/kg/day. After seven days of intravenous treatment, switching to 200 mg orally twice a day may be considered. Voriconazole has a milder side effect profile, and is much better tolerated than amphotericin B. The most frequent adverse effect is visual disturbances described as blurred vision, photophobia, and altered color perception. Liver function test abnormalities and skin reactions are less common side effects [42].

Posaconazole is another broad-spectrum triazole that is effective and safe as salvage therapy in patients with invasive aspergillosis refractory to standard antifungal therapy [43].

Echinocandin derivatives such as caspofungin, micafungin, and anidulafungin are effective agents in treatment of IPA refractory to standard treatment and can be used as second line agents or in combination therapy [36].

Surgical resection has a limited role in management of IPA patients. However, it should be considered in patients with massive hemoptysis, pulmonary lesions close to the great blood vessels or pericardium, or for resection of residual localized pulmonary lesions in patients with continuing immunosuppression [44].

Management of IPA is difficult, and prophylaxis is an important approach for those patients at increased risk. Avoiding hospitalization of patients in construction areas and use of high-efficiency particulate air (HEPA) filtration with or without laminar air flow ventilation has proven to be efficient [36]. Itraconazole is effective in preventing fungal infections in neutropenic patients and posaconazole is effective for prophylaxis against IPA in patients with severe GVHD and other hematological malignancies [45].

While A.fumigatus is the most common cause of IPA, there are increasing reports of IPA in cancer patients due to other species such as A.niger, A.terreus and A.flavus. Some of these species such as A. terreus and A. nidulans are resistant to amphotericin B. A. terreus is the second most common species isolated with frequency of around 23%. Risk factors and outcome for A. terreus infection are similar to those for A. fumigatus infection. However, A. terreus is significantly more likely to be nosocomial in origin, and more likely to be resistant to amphotericin B. New triazole antifungal agents such as voriconazole and posaconazole have significantly better efficacy against A. terreus [36].

Mucor

Mucormycosis is unusual fungal infection in immuno-compromised patients that its incidence is increasing. In allogeneic stem-cell transplant recipients, mucormycosis accounts for 8% of invasive fungal infections, and commonly occurs more than 3 months after transplantation. Mucormycosis has the tendency to invade blood vessels with thrombosis and tissue necrosis, and usually involves sino-pulmonary tree. Its dissemination to other organs is rare.

Direct histologic examination of the involved fluid or tissue as well as culture is the recommended diagnostic approach for mucormycosis. Lipid formulations of amphotericin B are the treatment of choice. Surgical debridement or removal of infected tissue is also recommended whenever feasible [46].

Acute Respiratory Failure

Acute respiratory failure may develop in the context of several complications of neutropenia. In patients with febrile neutropenia, lung involvement is seen in 20% of patients and 15% of them may develop acute respiratory event [47]. Worsening pneumonia secondary to bacterial or fungal infections may lead to acute respiratory failure. Sepsis and fluid overload are other factors that lead to acute respiratory failure. In this section we will discuss unique causes of acute respiratory failure in patients with neutropenia.

G-CSF Induced Pulmonary Toxicity

Human granulocyte colony stimulating factor (G-CSF) is an important regulatory cytokine that has the ability to stimulate neutrophil production. G-CSF is widely used in cancer patients to hasten recovery from chemotherapy induced neutropenia and to mobilize progenitor cells for hematopoietic stem cell transplantation. Side effects of G-CSF have been reported in 30% of patients. Pulmonary adverse effects range from cough, dyspnea, and pulmonary infiltrates to severe ARDS. In a meta-analysis 84 cases of G-CSF related pulmonary toxicity reviewed [48]. G-CSF related pulmonary toxicity patients divided into 3 different categories. First group were patients who developed pulmonary toxicity when G-CSF used alone (2 patients). In the second group, patients had pulmonary toxicity when G-CSF used in combination with other potentially pulmonary toxic agents (73 patients). Group 3 were patients who developed pulmonary toxicity during G-CSF enhanced neutropenia recovery (9 patients). Group 3 patients developed ARDS not before or after, but during recovery of neutropenia, which was defined as the 7 day period centered on the day neutrophil count rose to > 1000 cells/mm^3. All of patients in this group had clinically documented, and most of them had microbiologically documented pneumonia. There was one documented death in the third group. Influx of neutrophils to lungs, enhancing

TNF- alpha release by alveolar macrophages, and potentiation of lung injury caused by other factors such as chemotherapy or infection are possible mechanisms of acute lung injury in patients with G-CSF related pulmonary toxicity [48].

Engraftment Syndrome

Engraftment syndrome is a febrile syndrome specific to hematopoietic stem cell transplant recipients. Its incidence is 11%, and occurs more frequently after autologous HSCT, usually within 96 hours of engraftment [49]. Etiology of this syndrome is poorly understood. Release of proinflammatory cytokines during engraftment is postulated to play a principal role. The incidence and severity of engraftment syndrome increase with the use of G-CSF that regulates the production of cytokines (TNF-α, IL-1B, and IL-8), which increase alveolar permeability and neutrophil influx [49].

Specific criteria have been suggested for diagnosis of engraftment syndrome following HSCT. The major criteria are temperature ≥ 38.3C with no identifiable infectious etiology, erythrodermatous rash involving more than 25% of body surface area and not attributable to a medication, and noncardiogenic pulmonary edema manifested by diffuse pulmonary infiltrates consistent with the diagnosis and hypoxia (Figure 3). Minor criteria include hepatic dysfunction, renal insufficiency, weight gain ≥ 2.5% of baseline body weight, and transient encephalopathy unexplainable by other causes. Three major or two major and one or more minor criteria are needed for diagnosis of engraftment syndrome following HSCT [50].

Prognosis of engraftment syndrome is generally favorable. Mild cases are managed by supportive measures while strong consideration should be given to discontinue G-CSF. More severe cases, especially those with pulmonary involvement have dramatic response to systemic corticosteroids with improvement within the first day of treatment. Patients who require mechanical ventilation have the worst prognosis [50].

Acute Respiratory Distress Syndrome

Acute respiratory distress syndrome (ARDS) is the most serious cause of respiratory failure in neutropenic patients. ARDS usually complicates severe sepsis and pneumonia, and may develop following aspiration associated with mucositis, multiple blood transfusions, or chemotherapeutic agents. ARDS is defined by the presence of severe hypoxemia (PaO2/ FiO2 < 200), bilateral lung infiltrates consistent with pulmonary edema, and normal left ventricular function. Prognosis of ARDS has recently improved with advances in mechanical ventilation and ICU care. Lung protective ventilatory strategy is recommended in patients with or at risk of ARDS. A randomized controlled trial demonstrated that treating ARDS patients with lower tidal volume than traditional tidal volume will reduce the mortality by 22% [51] (Authors: this is irrelevant to the context. We are not talking about ARDS treatment.). There are only two studies that specifically address ARDS prognosis in neutropenic patients. In a prospective study, clinical features and outcome of 70 consecutive neutropenic cancer patients with ARDS were analyzed. Pulmonary system was the location of trigger in 43% and extra pulmonary in 30% patients. In 27% of patients etiology of ARDS was not determined [52].

The main etiologies of ARDS in these patients were sepsis (67%) and IA (11%). The 28 day mortality was 63%. Lobar ARDS, initial use of initial antibiotics active on difficult to treat bacteria such as pseudomonas, stenotrophomonas maltophilia, and extended- spectrum B- lactamase producing strains, and first line chemotherapy were factors independently associated with good prognosis. Markers of organ dysfunction (such as SAPS II), absence of neutropenia recovery and use of vasopressors during ICU stay was associated with higher mortality. This study also demonstrated that neither characteristics of underlying malignancy nor age were predictors of survival [52].

In another study, a cohort of consecutive neutropenic patients with hematologic malignancies were analyzed the risk factors for developing ARDS during recovery from neutropenia [53]. Seventy one patients who recovered from neutropenia were included in this retrospective analysis of a 6 years period, in which 38 (53.5%) of them were developed ARDS during recovery from neutropenia. Compared with non-ARDS patients, patients who experienced ARDS during neutropenia recovery were more likely to have pneumonia, be admitted to the ICU for respiratory failure, and receive mechanical ventilator therapy. The two groups had significantly different in-ICU mortality. The mortality for patients who developed ARDS during neutropenia recovery was 86.8% while patients without ARDS during neutropenia recovery had mortality of 51.5%. In multivariate analysis, occurrence of pneumonia during recovery from neutropenic period was the main risk factor associated with a marked increase in risk of ARDS. This study shows the importance of monitoring of patient respiratory status during neutrophil recovey and initiation of respiratory care as soon as possible in those patients who show signs of respiratory compromise [53].

Other Organ Considerations

C Difficile Colitis

Clostridium difficile colitis is another nosocomial infection that complicates clinical course of neutropenic patients secondary to chemotherapy or stem cell transplant. C difficile is a gram positive, spore forming anaerobe that colonizes gut following alteration of the normal flora with antibiotics. It causes antibiotic-associated colitis, which can range from a mild presentation to a fulminant course resulting in toxic mega colon and bowel perforation. Patients with hematopoetic stem cell transplant are at particularly high risk due to use of multiple antibiotics, prolonged hospital stay, neutropenia and immunossupression. In a retrospective study of 200 patients who had autologous peripheral blood stem cell transplant, 14 patients developed 15 instances (7.5%) of C difficile infection at a median follow up of 33 days [54].

In a retrospective study of 875 patients with myelosuppressive chemotherapy for hematologic malignancy and neutropenia, 7% of all patients developed C difficile associated diarrhea complicating myelosuppressive chemotherapy while 8.2% of this patients suffered from severe enterocolitis [55].

C difficile colitis commonly presents with watery diarrhea, low grade fever, leukocytosis, lower abdominal cramp and tenderness. In fulminant colitis, there will be severe abdominal pain and tenderness, distension, fever, hypovolemia, lactic acidosis and marked leukocytosis [56].

Diagnosis is made by a positive C difficile toxin in the presence of diarrhea. PCR for C difficile toxins A and B is highly sensitive and specific test with a rapid turnaround time and is preferred choice of study. Endoscopic study will show pseudo-membranes which are results of mucosal ulcerations covered by mucus and inflammatory cells. Endoscopic studies are not generally required except in cases where there is a high clinical suspicion for C difficile colitis with negative laboratory test, failure to respond to appropriate therapy or in atypical presentations [57].

Oral metronidazole or vancomycin for 10-14 days is the treatment of choice for C difficile colitis. Oral vancomycin is used as a first line agent in those with severe or recurrent disease and its efficacy is more than 90% [58].

There is also convincing evidence for the efficacy of duodenal infusion of donor feces in recurrent C difficile colitis as compared to oral vancomycin [59]. Surgical evaluation should be made in cases of fulminant C difficile colitis as colectomy could be life saving in such patients who are otherwise fit for surgery [60].

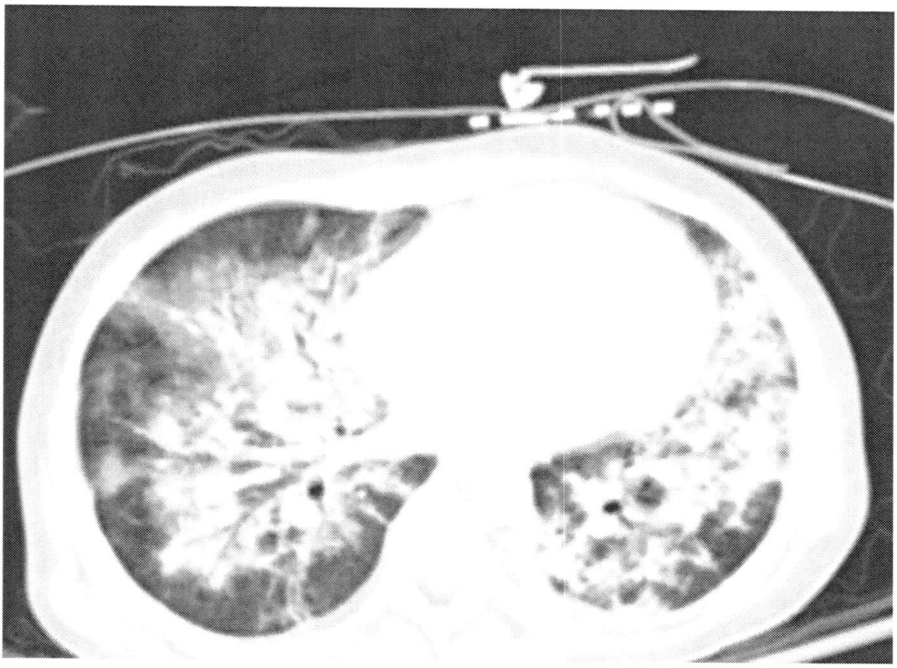

Figure 3. Chest CT image showing bilateral alveolar infiltrates of autologous HSCT recipient with engraftment syndrome.

Typhlitis (Neutropenic Enterocolitis)

Typhlitis is a unique and serious complication of neutropenia which is associated with a very high mortality. It should be considered in a neutropenic patient presenting with fever, abdominal pain and tenderness, with or without rebound tenderness. The pathophysiology of neutropenic enterocolitis involves mucosal injury from chemotherapy, neutropenia and impaired host defense. Histological examination may show transmural edema, mucosal ulceration and necrosis. Cecum is almost always involved with extension of inflammation to the terminal ileum and colon [61].

Presentation can be subtle and non specific or dramatic with signs of peritonitis, bowel perforation and sepsis. Imaging features, particularly computed tomography of the abdomen, suggestive of typhlitis include diffuse cecal wall thickening, intramural edema and inflammatory fat stranding along with the affected small bowel [62].

Management includes supportive care with bowel rest, intravenous hydration, total parentral nutrition and broad spectrum antimicrobials. In cases of uncontrolled bleeding, perforation and clinical deterioration despite medical therapy surgery is indicated. Use of granulocyte colony stimulating factor to hasten neutrophil recovery is also recommended [61].

Finally patients with neutropenia and severe sepsis with multi-organ failure need several additional supports. Correction of coagulopathy in patients with disseminated intravascular coagulation, renal replacement therapy for those with acute renal failure, ensuing complications not amenable to medical management, and evaluation and management of neurologic abnormalities are some of those supportive measures.

Supportive Care in Neutropenic Fever

Granulocyte Colony Stimulating Factor (G-CSF)

Studies have shown that G-CSF may reduce duration of neutropenia as well as risk of neutropenic fever. G-CSF is recommended in chemotherapy regimens with risk of neutropenic fever exceeding 20% and in those with high risk features for chemotherapy induced neutropenia (old age, previous history of neutropenia and use of myelotoxic agents) [63-64].

G-CSF has also been routinely used in post-transplant setting to facilitate neutrophil recovery [65]. However, role of G-CSF in patients with febrile neutropenia is not well defined and several studies have showed controversive results. According to the American Society Clinical Oncology, currently available data is not enough to support routine use of G-CSF in patients with febrile neutropenia. Nevertheless, G-CSF should be considered in patients with febrile neutropenia and high risk features such as profound neutropenia ($< 100/mm^3$), expected prolonged neutropenia (more than 10 days), age > 65years, and manifestations of severe sepsis [63].

Granulocyte Transfusion

Granulocyte transfusion in patients with severe infection has been studied for several decades with disappointing outcomes in earlier investigations. More recent data showed benefit for a subgroup of neutropenic patients with severe, uncontrolled infection. Granulocyte transfusion benefits were also seen in patients with severe uncontrolled fungal infection [66]. It should be noted that graft versus host disease is a potentially serious complication of granulocyte transfusion in patients who had stem cell transplant. In addition, studies have shown that patient's outcome is depending on underlying disease process and recovery of their own neutrophils rather than granulocyte transfusion [67-68].

Neutropenic Precautions

Several infection control measures have been attempted in patients with neutropenia even though there is no evidence of clear benefit. A prospective study failed to show protective effect of strict infection control measures (caps, masks, gown and gloves) on clonal spread of coagulase negative staphylococci colonizing central catheters in neutropenic patients with cancer [69]. On the other hand, hand washing is a simple method that has been shown to reduce transmission of nosocomial infections [70].

Conclusion

Neutropenia is an important complication of chemotherapy, stem cell transplant and infections. Patients with neutropenia may develop severe complications that require immediate attention and commonly care in the intensive care units. Clinical course of infections in neutropenic patients may be atypical and rapidly progressive. In addition, neutropenic patients may have infections from unusual bacterial and fungal organisms, which can pose a diagnostic and therapeutic challenge. Noninfectious causes of fever in neutropenic patients including engraftment syndrome should also be considered and properly treated. Multidisciplinary approach in the care of these critically ill patients that includes the intensivist and hematologist is needed and involvement of other specialties is strongly recommended. The same guidelines for care of critically ill neutropenic patients should be followed as those developed for other critically ill patients. These include following the surviving sepsis guidelines and lung protective strategies for patients with acute lung injury or ARDS. Supportive and prophylactic measures are vital in these patients. Simple infection control measures including proper hand washing have been shown to be effective in reducing transmission of nosocomial infections in neutropenic patients.

References

[1] Dale D. C., Cottle T. E., Fier C. J. et al. Severe chronic neutropenia: treatment and follow-up of patients in the Severe Chronic Neutropenia International Registry. *American Journal of Hematology.* 2003 Feb; 72(2):82-93.

[2] Van der Klauw M. M., Goudsmit R., Halie M. R. et al. A population-based case-cohort study of drug-associated agranulocytosis. *Arch Intern Med.* 1999; 159(4):369.

[3] Keng M. K., Sekeres M. A. Febrile neutropenia in hematologic malignancies. *Curr Hematol Malig Rep.* 2013 Dec; 8(4):370-8.

[4] Freifeld A. G., Bow E. J., Sepkowitz K. A. et al. Clinical Practice Guideline for the Use of Antimicrobial Agents in Neutropenic Patients with Cancer: 2010. Update by the Infectious Diseases Society of America. *Clin Infect Dis.* 2011 Feb 15; 52 (4): 56-93.

[5] Nakagawa Y., Suzuki K., Ohta K. Prospective randomized study of cefepime, panipenem, or meropenem monotherapy for patients with hematological disorders and febrile neutropenia. *J Infect Chemother,* 2012 Feb; 19(1):103-11.

[6] Courtney D. M., Aldeen A. Z., Gorman S. M. et al. Cancer-Associated Neutropenic Fever: Clinical Outcome and Economic Costs of Emergency Department Care. *The Oncologist* 2007; 12:1019-1026.

[7] Kosmidis C., Chandrasekar P: Management of gram-positive bacterial infections in patients with cancer. *Leukemia & Lymphoma,* January 2012; 53(1): 8-18.

[8] Matsuoka H., Tsukamoto A., Shirahashi A. et al. Efficacy of intravenous ciprofloxacin in patients with febrile neutropenia refractory to initial therapy. *Leukemia & Lymphoma,* August 2006; 47(8): 1618- 1623.

[9] Jaksic B., Martinelli G., Perez-Oteyza J. et al. Efficacy and safety of linezolid compared with vancomycin in a randomized, double-blind

study of febrile neutropenic patients with cancer. *Clin Infect Dis.* 2006 Mar 1; 42 (5):597-607.

[10] Ru¨ ping M., Vehreschild J., Cornely O., Antifungal treatment strategies in high risk patients. *Mycose,* May 2008, 51 (Suppl. 2), 46-51.

[11] Cordonnier C., Pautas C., Maury S. et al. Empirical versus Preemptive Antifungal Therapy for High-Risk, Febrile, Neutropenic Patients: A Randomized, Controlled Trial. *Clinical Infectious Diseases.* 2009; 48:1042-51.

[12] Ito J. I., Kriengkauykiat J., Dadwal S. S., Arfons L. M., Lazarus H. M. Approaches to the early treatment of invasive fungal infection. *Leuk Lymphoma.* 2010 Sep; 51 (9): 1623-31.

[13] Bone R. C., Balk R. A., Cerra F. B. et al. Definitions for sepsis and organ failure and guidelines for the use of innovative therapies in sepsis. The ACCP/SCCM Consensus Conference Committee. American College of Chest Physicians/ Society of Critical Care Medicine. *Chest* June 1992; 101(6):1644-1655.

[14] Michael Darmon, Elie Azoulay, Corinne Alberti et al. Impact of neutropenia duration on short-term mortality in neutropenic critically ill cancer patients. *Intensive Care Med* (2002) 28:1775-1780.

[15] Legrand M., Max A., Peigne V. et al. Survival in neutropenic patients with severe sepsis or septic shock. *Crit Care Med* 2012 Jan; (40) 1: 43-9.

[16] Nguyen H. B., Corbett S. W., Menes K., Early goal-directed therapy, corticosteroid, and recombinant human activated protein C for the treatment of severe sepsis and septic shock in the emergency department. *Acad Emerg Med.* 2006 Jan; 13(1): 109-13.

[17] Rivers E., Nguyen B., Havstad S. et al. Early Goal-Directed Therapy Collaborative Group. Early goal-directed therapy in the treatment of severe sepsis and septic shock. *N Engl J Med.* 2001 Nov 8; 345(19):1368-7.

[18] Kumar A., Roberts D., Wood K. E. et al. M. Duration of hypotension before initiation of effective antimicrobial therapy is the critical determinant of survival in human septic shock. *Crit Care Med.* 2006 Jun; 34(6):1589-96.

[19] Jones A., Focht A., Horton J. et al. Prospective External Validation of the Clinical Effectiveness of an Emergency Department-Based Early Goal-Directed Therapy Protocol for Severe Sepsis and Septic Shock. *CHEST.* August 2007; 132(2):425-432).

[20] Trzeciak S., Dellinger R. P., Chansky M. E. et al. Serum lactate as a predictor of mortality in patients with infection. *Intensive Care Med* (2007) 33(6):970–977.

[21] Hanzelka K. M., Yeung S. C., Chisholm G. et al. Implementation of modified early-goal directed therapy for sepsis in the emergency center of a comprehensive cancer center. *Support Care Cancer.* 2013 Mar; 21(3): 727-34.

[22] Bodro M., Sabé N., Gomila A. et al. Risk Factors, Clinical Characteristics, and Outcomes Invasive Fungal Infections in Solid Organ Transplant Recipients. *Transplant Proc.* 2012 Nov; 44(9):2682-5.

[23] Ullmann A. J., Akova M, R. Herbrecht R. et al. ESCMID guideline for the diagnosis and management of Candida diseases 2012: Adults with hematological malignancies and after hematopoietic stem cell transplantation (HCT); *Clinical Microbiology and Infection,* Volume 18 Supplement 7, December 2012.

[24] Pappas P. G., Kauffman C. A., Andes D., et al. Clinical practice guidelines for the management of candidiasis: 2009 update by the Infections Diseases Society of America. *Clin Infect Dis* 2009; 48:503.

[25] Lambourne J., Agranoff D., Herbrecht R. et al. Association of mannose-binding lectin deficiency with acute invasive aspergillosis in immunocompromised patients. *Clin Infect Dis.* 2009; 49(10):1486.

[26] Gerson S. L., Talbot G. H., Hurwitz S., Strom B. L., Lusk E. J., Cassileth P. A. Prolonged granulocytopenia: the major risk factor for invasive pulmonary aspergillosis in patients with acute leukemia. *Ann Intern Med.* 1984 Mar; 100(3):345-51.

[27] Marr K. A., Carter R. A., Boeckh M., Martin P., Corey L. Invasive Aspergillosis in allogeneic stem cell transplant recipients: changes in epidemiology and risk factors. *Blood* 2002; 100 (13): 4358-66.

[28] Fukuda T., Boeckh M., Carter R. A. et al. Risks and outcomes of invasive fungal infections in recipients of allogeneic hematopoietic stem cell transplants after nonmyeloablative conditioning. *Blood* 2003; 102(3):827-33.

[29] Ruhnke M., Bohme A., Buchheidt D. et al. Diagnosis of invasive fungal infections in hematology and oncology: Guidelines of the Infectious Diseases Working Party (AGIHO) of the German Society of Hematology and Oncology (DGHO). *Ann Hematol* 2003; 82 Suppl 2:S141-8.

[30] Chamilos G., Luna M., Lewis R. E. et al. Invasive fungal infections in patients with hematologic malignancies in a tertiary care cancer center:

an autopsy study over a 15-year period (1989-2003). *Haematologica* 2006; 91(7):986-9.

[31] Kuhlman J. E., Fishman E. K., Siegelman S. S. Invasive pulmonary aspergillosis in acute leukemia: characteristic findings on CT, the CT halo sign, and the role of CT in early diagnosis. *Radiology* 1985; 157(3):611-4.

[32] Caillot D., Casasnovas O., Bernard A. et al. Improved management of invasive pulmonary aspergillosis in neutropenic patients using early thoracic computed tomographic scan and surgery. *J Clin Oncol* 1997; 15(1):139-47.

[33] Greene R. The radiological spectrum of pulmonary aspergillosis. *Med Mycol* 2005; 43 Suppl 1:S147-54.

[34] Horvath J. A., Dummer S. The use of respiratory-tract cultures in the diagnosis of invasive pulmonary aspergillosis. *Am J Med* 1996; 100(2):171-8.

[35] Yu V. L., Muder R. R., Poorsattar A. Significance of isolation of Aspergillus from the respiratory tract in diagnosis of invasive pulmonary aspergillosis. Results from a three-year prospective study. *Am J Med* 1986; 81(2):249-54.

[36] Kousha M., Tadi R., Soubani A. O. Pulmonary aspergillosis: A clinical review. *Eur Respir Rev.* 2011 Sep 1; 20(121):156-74.

[37] Pfeiffer C. D., Fine J. P., Safdar N. Diagnosis of invasive aspergillosis using a galactomannan assay: a meta-analysis. *Clin Infect Dis* 2006;42(10):1417-727.

[38] Marr K. A., Balajee S. A., McLaughlin L., Tabouret M., Bentsen C., Walsh T. J. Detection of galactomannan antigenemia by enzyme immunoassay for the diagnosis of invasive aspergillosis: Variables that affect performance. *J Infect Dis 2004;* 190(3):641-9.

[39] Klont R. R., Mennink-Kersten M. A., Verweij P. E. Utility of Aspergillus antigen detection in specimens other than serum specimens. *Clin Infect Dis* 2004; 39(10):1467-74.

[40] Hizel K., Kokturk N., Kalkanci A., Ozturk C., Kustimur S., Tufan M. Polymerase chain reaction in the diagnosis of invasive aspergillosis. *Mycoses* 2004; 47(7):338-42.

[41] Obayashi T., Yoshida M., Mori T. et al. Plasma (1- > 3)-beta-D-glucan measurement in diagnosis of invasive deep mycosis and fungal febrile episodes. *Lancet* 1995;345(8941):17-20.

[42] Johnson L. B., Kauffman C. A. Voriconazole: A new triazole antifungal agent. *Clin Infect Dis* 2003; 36(5):630-7.

[43] Segal B. H., Barnhart L. A., Anderson V. L., Walsh T. J., Malech H. L., Holland S. M. Posaconazole as salvage therapy in patients with chronic granulomatous disease and invasive filamentous fungal infection. *Clin Infect Dis* 2005; 40(11):1684-8.

[44] Reichenberger F., Habicht J., Kaim A. et al. Lung resection for invasive pulmonary aspergillosis in neutropenic patients with hematologic diseases. *Am J Respir Crit Care Med* 1998; 158(3):885-90.

[45] Ullmann A. J., Lipton J. H., Vesole D. H. et al. Posaconazole or fluconazole for prophylaxis in severe graft-versus-host disease. *N Engl J Med* 2007;356(4):335-47.

[46] Lanternier F., Sun., Ribaud P. et al. Mucormycosis in organ and stem cell transplant recipients. *Clin Infect Dis.* 2012 Jun; 54(11):1629-36.

[47] Rossini F., Verga M., Pioltelli P., Giltri G., Sancassani V., Pogliani E. M., Corneo G. Incidence and outcome of pneumonia in patients with acute leukemia receiving first induction therapy with anthracycline-containing regimens. *Haematologica.* 2000 Dec; 85(12):1255-60.

[48] Azoulay E., Attalah H., Harf A., Schlemmer B., Delclaux C. Granulocyte colony stimulating factor or neutrophil-induced pulmonary toxicity: Myth or reality? Systematic review of clinical case reports and experimental data. *Chest 2001;* 120(5):1695-701.

[49] Soubani A. O., Pandya C. M. The spectrum of noninfectious pulmonary complications following hematopoietic stem cell transplantation. *Hematol Oncol Stem Cell Ther.* 2010; 3(3):143-57.

[50] Spitzer T. R. Engraftment syndrome following hematopoietic stem cell transplantation. *Bone Marrow Transplant* 2001; 27(9):893-8.

[51] The Acute Respiratory Distress Syndrome Network: Ventilation with lower tidal volumes as compared with traditional tidal volumes for acute lung injury and the acute respiratory distress syndrome. *N Engl J Med.* 2000 May 4; 342(18):1301–1308.

[52] Mokart D., van Craenenbroeck T., Lambert J. et al. Prognosis of acute respiratory distress syndrome in neutropenic cancer patients. *Eur Respi J.* 2012 Jul; 40(1):169-76.

[53] Rhee C. K., Kang J. Y., Kim Y. H. et al. Risk factors for acute respiratory distress syndrome during neutropenia recovery in patients with hematologic malignancies. *Crit Care.* 2009; 13(6):R173.

[54] Bilgrami S., Feingold J. M., Dorsky D. et al. Incidence and outcome of Clostridium difficile infection following autologous peripheral blood stem cell transplantation. *Bone Marrow Transplantation.* 1999 May; 23(10): 1039-1042.

[55] Gorschluter M., Glasmacher A., Hahn C. et al. Clostridium difficile Infection in Patients with Neutropenia. *Clinical Infectious Diseases* 2001; 33:786-91.

[56] Rubin M. S., Bodenstein L. E., Kent K. C., Severe Clostridium difficile colitis. *Dis Colon Rectum.* 1995; 38(4):350.

[57] Triadafilopoulos G., Hallstone A. E., Acute abdomen as the first presentation of pseudomembraneous colitis. *Gastroenterology.* 1991 Sep; 101(3):685-91.

[58] Vicki R. Kee, Clostridium Difficile Infection in Older Adults: A Review and Update on Its Management. *The American Journal of Geriatric Pharmacotherapy,* Feb 2012, 10(1).

[59] Van Nood E., Vrieze A., Nieuwdorp M. et al. Duodenal Infusion of Donor Feces for Recurrent Clostridium difficile. *N Engl J Med* 2013; 368:407-415.

[60] Stewart D. B., Hollenbeak C. S., Wilson M. Z. Is colectomy for fulminant c difficile colitis life saving? A systematic review. *Colorectal* Dis. 2013 Jan 25.

[61] Marta L. Davila ;Neutropenic enterocolitis. *Current Opinion in Gastroenterology* 2006, 22:44-47.

[62] Ullery B. W., Pieracci F. M., Rodney J. R., Barie P. S. Neutropenic enterocolitis. *Surg Infect (Larchmt).* 2009 Jun; 10(3):307-14.

[63] Smith T. J., Khatcheressian J., Lyman G. H. et al. 2006 update of recommendations for the use of white blood cell growth factors: an evidence-based clinical practice guideline. *J Clin Oncol.* 2006; 24(19):3187.

[64] Aapro M. S., Bohlius J., Cameron D. A. et al. 2010 update of EORTC guidelines for the use of granulocyte-colony stimulating factor to reduce the incidence of chemotherapy-induced febrile neutropenia in adult patients with lymphoproliferative disorders and solid tumors. *Eur J Cancer.* 2011 Jan; 47(1):8-32.

[65] Taylor K. M., Jagannath S., Spitzer G. et al. Recombinant human granulocyte colony-stimulating factor hastens granulocyte recovery after high-dose chemotherapy and autologous bone marrow transplantation in Hodgkin's disease. *JCO* December 1989 vol. 7 no. 12 1791-1799.

[66] Cesaro S., Chinello P., Silvestro G. et al. Granulocyte transfusions from G-CSF-stimulated donors for the treatment of severe infections in neutropenic pediatric patients with onco-hematological diseases. *Support Care Cancer* (2003) 11: 101-106.

[67] Ehab Atallah and Charles A. Schiffer: Granulocyte transfusion. *Current Opinion in Hematology* 2006, 13:45-49.

[68] Marfin A. A., Price T. H. Granulocyte Transfusion Therapy. *J Intensive Care Med.* 2013 Aug 5. (Epub ahead of print).

[69] Van Pelt a C, Nouwen a J, Lugtenburg E. et al. Strict infection control measures do not prevent clonal spread of coagulase negative staphylococci colonizing central venous catheters in neutropenic hemato-oncologic patients. *FEMS Immunology and Medical Microbiology*. 2003 Sep 22; 38(2): 153-158.

[70] Pittet D, Hugonnet S, Harbarth S. et al. Effectiveness of a hospital-wide programme to improve compliance with hand hygiene. *Lancet* 2000; 356: 1307-12.

Index

A

B

C

D

E

F

G

H

I

J

K

L

M

Q

R

S

T

U

V

W

Y

Z